The Anti-Inflammatory Diet Cookbook

100 Recipes To Prevent and Reverse Full Spectrum Of Inflammatory Symptoms and Diseases

LESLIE PHILIPS

ISBN-13: 978-1719345712

ISBN-10: 1719345716

DEDICATION

To all who desire to live life to the fullest!

TABLE OF CONTENT

INTRODUCTION

On the whole, the pain, swelling, heat and local redness on the body's surface when infected or injured are all indications of inflammation. When the body is infected or injured, inflammation brings more immune activity and nourishment to the injured spot, serving as the foundation for the body's healing response, alerting our body to something wrong. Then again, any inflammation that is not nourishing the body, or any persistent inflammation will cause illnesses and damage to the body. It is no longer news that most serious sicknesses, which include Alzheimer's diseases, several cancers and heart disease, can be linked to chronic inflammation. Toxic exposures (such as tobacco smoke), genetic tendencies, lack of exercise and stress can all add up to cause chronic inflammation. Chronic inflammation is an indication of a severe underlying problem that spells trouble if left unchecked.

The Anti-Inflammatory Diet is not your regular diet, it is a diet based on the methodical understanding of choosing and preparing anti-inflammatory foods that can best sustain optimal health. Certain foods are anti-inflammatory and can be used to control the inflammatory process, reduce disease susceptibility and contain inflammation in a very effective way. The anti-inflammatory diet also supplies protective phytonutrients, essential fatty acids dietary fiber, minerals, plentiful vitamins and steady energy.

Your way of life is equally as important as your dietary choices. Reaching excellent health calls for a suitable anti-inflammatory diet, avoiding unwarranted stress, habitual exercise {30-60 minutes, 4 or more times weekly} and getting enough sleep. The anti-inflammatory diet with some basic daily-life changes will help you prevent the risk of severe health problems caused by inflammation. You can enjoy a stress-free and better life with little or no illnesses.

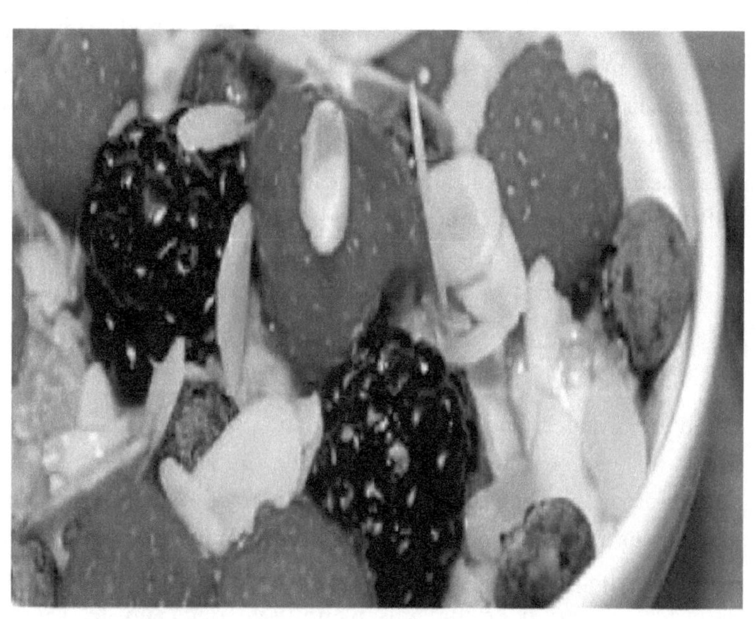

What is Inflammation

Inflammation characterizes a vital survival system that helps the body battle off unfriendly microbes and restores damaged tissue. Studies show that inflammation, partly assisted by some other factors such as an inactive daily life, smoking and obesity, contributes to an array of illnesses. The recognizable feeling of heat, swelling, redness and pain produced from an infection or injury are features of the inflammatory process. Inflammation is in two forms, which include 1) acute inflammation 2) chronic inflammation.

Acute Inflammation

Acute inflammation starts out very quickly within a short time, but this type of inflammation is generally transitory. When injured or infected, this inflammation process is activated to attack hostile microbes, remove dead cells and mend any damaged cells. This process restores the infected or injured site to a steady form, and inflammation disappears after some hours or days.

Chronic Inflammation

Chronic inflammation starts out in the same way as acute inflammation, but metamorphoses into a persistent condition. In this state, the immune system response becomes unsuccessful at removing the problem for months or even years. Then again, chronic inflammation may remain active even after correcting the initial injury or infection. Also, low-level inflammation can be activated even without apparent disease or injury. If these low-level inflammations are not corrected, the immune system will instruct white blood cells to assault healthy tissues and organs that are close by, and these attacks on healthy tissues and organs sets up a chronic inflammatory progression that serves as the basis for many severe diseases of today, such as Alzheimer's, asthma, diabetes, heart disease and rheumatoid arthritis.

Family history, diet and lifestyle choices are factors that assist partly in the medical conditions and disease caused by chronic inflammation. Chronic inflammation can be successfully controlled, prevented and reversed by making few lifestyle changes and eating anti-inflammatory foods.

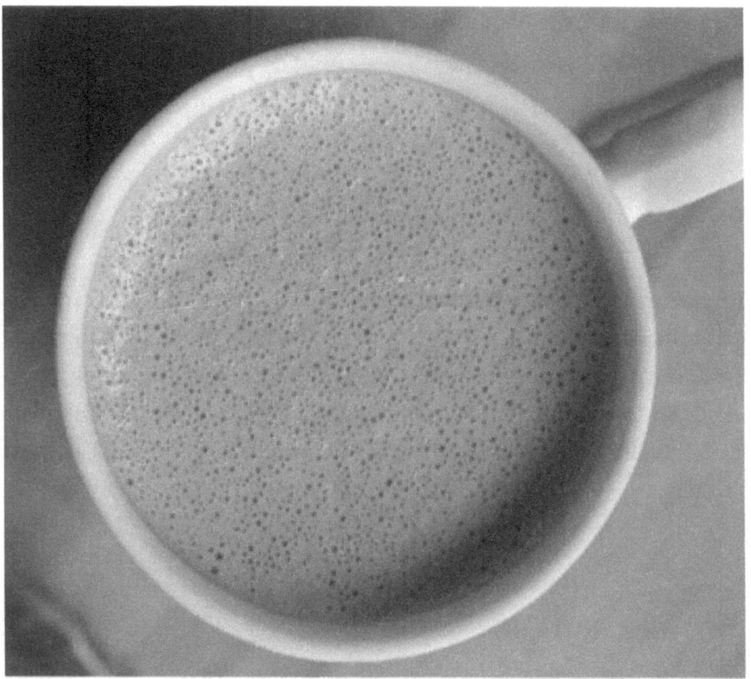

The Anti-Inflammatory Diet

The anti-inflammatory diet is not completely a set of rules or an anti-inflammatory eating plan. Unlike most regular health or weight loss diets around, the anti-inflammatory diet is a pretty straightforward diet. There are several foods that can be eaten on the diet and how much can be eaten is very flexible. It is recommended to eat more foods that fight inflammation and less of foods that cause inflammation. Theoretically, the Whole30 diets, Mediterranean diet and many other diets can be categorized as anti-inflammatory diets even though they have their differences.

Kick Start Guide

There are several benefits to eating anti-inflammatory foods, including a reduced heart disease risk, weight loss and more energy. While starting out on the diet, it is important to seek the advice of a nutritionist or doctor for an eating-plan that is best suitable for you. The anti-inflammatory diet is not suitable for a diabetic, an expectant or nursing mother. If you experience chronic inflammation, such as rheumatoid arthritis or psoriasis, then your symptoms can be managed with an anti-inflammatory diet.

Your dietary choices play a major part in the reduction and control of long-term disease risk.

What and What Not to Eat

An anti-inflammatory diet focuses on eating more healthy fats, low-fat dairy, veggies, fruits, lean proteins and whole grains. There are several nutritious and scrumptious food options on the diet. Consumption of foods that are connected to inflammation, which includes, red meat, high-glycemic index foods (such as pasta and white bread made from white flour), too much sugar, fried and processed foods should be drastically reduced or totally avoided.

Anti-Inflammation Diet Tips

Several existing recipes can be adapted to the anti-inflammatory diet by following these tips:

- Consume veggies and fruits in large quantities.
- Drastically reduce or totally eliminate eating junks, fast foods, fried and processed foods.
- Eat more whole fresh foods as you can.
- Eat from an assortment of food options.

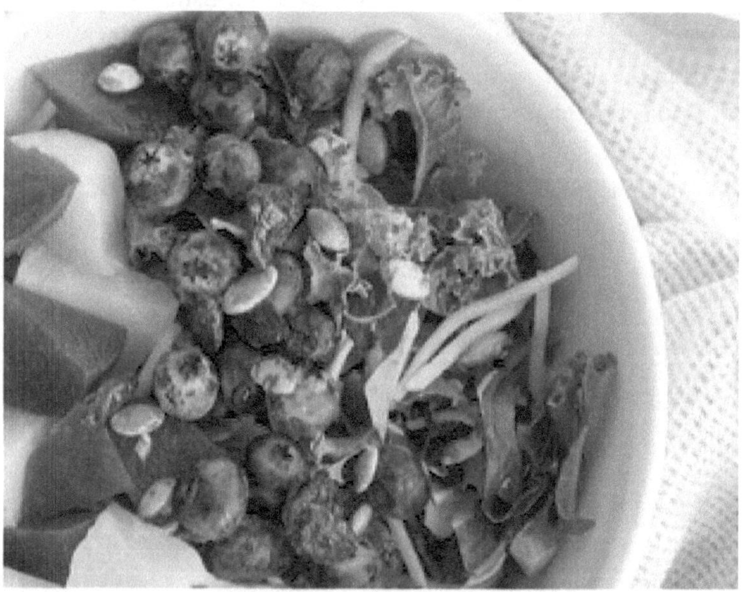

Daily Caloric Distribution

A large number of adults eat between 2000-3000 calories every day- with men needing more calories than the women. Bigger and more active people need additional calories per day, while smaller and less active people need a smaller amount of calories per day. When you eat the right amount of calories needed for your activity level, your body weight will be balanced. The calories consumed from each food class based on their nutrient properties should be as like this: Carbs 40%-50%, Protein 20%-30%, and Fat 30% of the daily caloric intake. Ensure each meal is loaded with protein, fat and carbs in their right proportions.

Carbs

Adult men should eat 240-300g of carbs per day on a 2000 calorie per day diet, while women should eat 160-200g daily. Carbohydrates consumed should be less-processed and less-refined with a low glycemic load. Avoid eating foods that are loaded with sugar and wheat flour, including many packaged snack foods (like pretzels and chips) and bread. Also, avoid foods that are made with high fructose corn syrup. Consume more carbohydrates that are whole grains, like bulgur wheat and brown rice. Consume more sweet potatoes, winter squashes and beans. Pasta should be cooked al dente and eaten in moderate amounts.

Protein

If you have autoimmune disease, allergies, kidney or liver problems, you should eat less protein. On a 2000 calorie per day diet, you should consume 80-120g protein. Eat less of animal protein such as red meat, poultry, not including fish. Eat more high quality yogurt, natural cheese and fish. Consume more veggie protein, like beans (especially soybeans)

Fat

Foods loaded with saturated fat should be much reduced such as, foods made with palm kernel oil, fatty meats, unskinned chicken and turkey, high fat cheese, cream and butter. 600 of 2000 calorie per day diet can come from fat, approximately 67grams fat. Cook more with extra-virgin olive oil. Keep away from mixed vegetable oils, cotton seed oil, corn oil, and the regular sunflower and safflower oils. Keep away from foods made with partially hydrogenated oils. Keep away from foods that have vegetable shortening and margarine as ingredients and avoid them completely. Consume more almonds, cashews, walnuts and avocados. Eat nut-based butters made from almonds, cashews and walnuts.

Omega 3 Fatty Acids

Eat freshly ground flaxseeds and hemp seeds, omega-3 fortified eggs, butterfish, sablefish, herring, sardines packed in olive oil or water and canned sockeye or frozen wild or fresh salmon. You can also take 2-3g daily dosage of fish oil supplements (with DHA & EPA provision).

Phytonutrients

Phytonutrients wholly protects you from environmental toxins, age-linked diseases, which include neurodegenerative disease, cancer and cardiovascular disease. Eat foods loaded with phytonutrients, such as mushrooms, veggies and fruits. Eat dark leafy greens, yellow fruits, oranges, tomatoes and berries. Make sure your food is produced organically without pesticides and other harmful chemicals. Habitually eat more soy foods, cruciferous veggies (cabbage and its relatives). Drink good quality oolong, green or white tea instead of coffee. If you have to take alcohol, take red wine preferably. Eat plain dark chocolate (70% or more cocoa content) in moderate amounts.

Fiber

Consume around 40g of fiber in a day. Eat more whole grains, veggies (particularly beans) and fruits (particularly berries). Make sure any ready-made cereal gives you about 4-5g bran/1-oz. serving.

Water

Stay hydrated during the day with drinks that are mostly water, such as sparkling water with lemon, extremely diluted fruit juice and tea. Take pure water. Avoid drinking contaminated water or chlorine tasting water.

Vitamins and Minerals

For a diet that is loaded in minerals and vitamins, eat a diet that is high in fresh whole foods with surplus veggies and fruits. You can also supplement your diet.

Prevent and reverse inflammatory symptoms and diseases by getting started on the anti-inflammatory diet journey with a variety of foods to choose from. Eat your way to health and longevity.

Anti-Inflammatory Recipes To Prevent and Reverse Inflammatory Symptoms and Diseases

Breakfast Recipes

Avocado Egg Toast

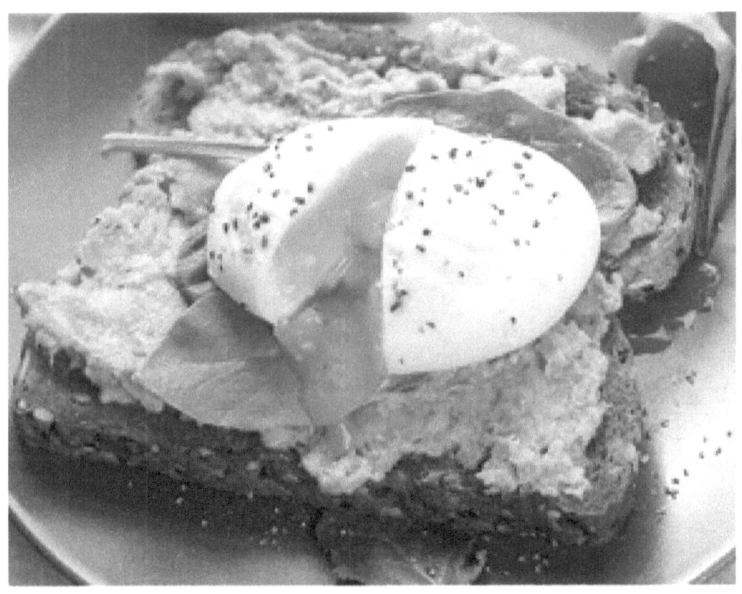

Preparation Time: 5 minutes

Cook Time: 8 minutes

Serves: 1 serving

Ingredients

1½ teaspoon ghee

2 toasted gluten-free bread slice

1 handful spinach

½ avocado

Red pepper flakes

1 (scrambled or poached) egg

Instructions

1. Top the toasted bread slice with ghee.

2. Spread avocado on the ghee coated toast.

3. Top toast with scrambled or poached egg and fresh spinach leaves.

4. Garnish toast with a liberal sprinkle of red pepper flakes.

5. Cover open faced sandwich with the second toasted bread slice.

Delicious Breakfast Muffins

Preparation Time: 10 minutes

Cook Time: 20 minutes

Serves: 12 muffins

Ingredients

1/2 cup flaxseed meal

1/2 cup almond meal

1/2 cup spelt flour

1/2 cup oat bran

1/3 cup brown sugar

1/2 cup flour, whole wheat

1 tsp baking powder

2 tsps baking soda

1 egg white

1 egg

1/2 cup applesauce

3/4 cup buttermilk

1 cup (chopped) walnuts

2 (mashed) ripe bananas

1/2 cup raisins

Instructions

1. Heat up oven to 350°F.

2. Prepare a well-greased 12-tin muffin pan with butter.

3. Add baking powder, baking soda, brown sugar, whole wheat flour, spelt flour, oat bran, flaxseed meal and almond milk into a big bowl and mix until combined.

4. Add egg white and egg into a small bowl and beat until combined.

5. Add bananas, applesauce, buttermilk and the egg mixture into the flour mixture.

6. Stir flour mixture until combined but do not over-mix.

7. Add raisins and walnuts into the mixture and stir until evenly distributed.

8. Scoop batter into the prepared muffin tins and transfer into the preheated oven.

9. Bake muffins for 18-20 minutes, until set.

Cheesy Beet Open Faced Sandwich

Preparation Time: 5 minutes

Cook Time: 20 minutes

Serves: 4 servings

Ingredients

1 tbsp olive oil + more for garnish

4 (scrubbed) small red beets

¼ tsp salt

1 tbsp brown rice vinegar

4 oz. (at room temperature) soft goat cheese

Ground pepper, as needed

4 (1/2" thick) slices {lightly toasted} crusty whole-grain bread

2 tbsps milk

Garnish with

Fresh thyme

Instructions

1. Fit a steamer basket into a big saucepan and add just 1" of water.

2. Bring water to boiling.

3. Add beets into the boiling water, place lid over saucepan and steam for 10-15 minutes until beets are softened.

4. Remove beets, place on a cutting board and let sit until wholly cool to touch.

5. Use kitchen paper to rub off beet skin, slice beets into wedges and place in a bowl.

6. Sprinkle pepper, salt, and oil over beets and toss until combined.

7. Add milk and goat cheese into a fairly big bowl and stir until a smooth consistency is reached.

8. Sprinkle milk mixture with pepper.

9. Spread about 2 tbsps of the milk cheese mixture on each toasted bread slice, topped with some of the beets.

10. Garnish sandwich with thyme, if desired.

Almond Blueberry Chia Pudding

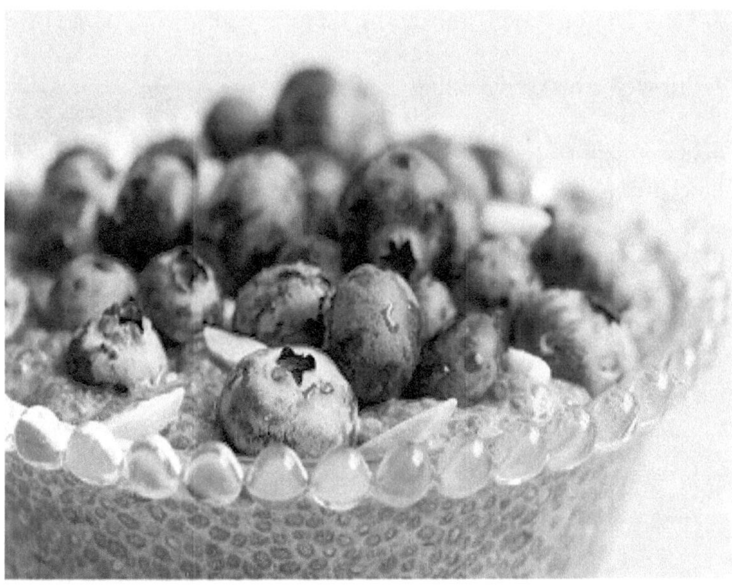

Preparation Time: 10 minutes

Cook Time: 0 minutes

Serves: 1 serving

Ingredients

2 tbsps chia seeds

½ cup coconut milk, unsweetened

1/3 tsp almond extract

2 tsps honey

1 tbsp (divided) slivered almonds, toasted

½ cup (divided) fresh blueberries

Instructions

1. Add almond extract, honey, chia and coconut milk into a small bowl.

2. Stir mixture until combined.

3. Place lid over bowl, transfer into a refrigerator for 8 hours or more.

4. Stir well after refrigerating.

5. Scoop half of the chia pudding into a bowl and top with almonds and blueberries.

6. Add the remaining chia pudding into the bowl, topped with the remaining almonds and blueberries.

7. Serve and enjoy.

Latte Overnight Oats with Almond milk and Green Tea

Preparation Time: 10 minutes

Cook Time: 0 minutes

Serves: 2 servings

Ingredients

1 tbsp chia seeds

1 cup rolled oats, old-fashioned

1 cup baby spinach, packed

1 tbsp hemp seeds

½ cup almond milk, unsweetened

1 cup (cooled to room temp) strong green tea

¼ tsp cinnamon

3 tbsps (soaked overnight in water) cashews

2 (pitted) medjool dates

½ tsp vanilla

Top with (If desired)

Bananas, sliced

Fresh berries

Cashews

Instructions

1. Add hemp seeds, chia seeds and oats into a fairly big bowl and combine.

2. Drain the soaked cashews.

3. Add cashews and every other remaining ingredient into a high speed blender.

TIP: Do not pour the oat mixture and the toppings into the blender.

4. Blend mixture until a smooth consistency is reached.

5. Pour the blended mixture into the oat mixture and combine.

6. Place lid over bowl and refrigerate overnight.

7. Split oats evenly into 2 serving bowls.

8. Top overnight oat with berries, bananas and seeds.

Matcha Banana Green Smoothie Bowl

Preparation Time: 10 minutes

Cook Time: 0 minutes

Serves: 1 serving

Ingredients

½ cup sliced peaches, frozen

½ cup sliced banana, frozen

½ cup almond milk, unsweetened

1 cup fresh spinach

1½ tsps matcha tea powder

5 tbsps (divided) almonds, slivered

½ ripe (diced) kiwi

1 tsp maple syrup

Instructions

1. Add maple syrup, matcha powder, 3 tbsps almonds, almond milk, spinach, peaches and banana into a high speed electric blender.

2. Blend mixture until a very smooth consistency is reached.

3. Pour blended smoothie into a bowl, topped with the remaining 2 tbsps slivered almonds and kiwi.

4. Serve and enjoy.

Delicious Whole-Grain Amaranth Porridge

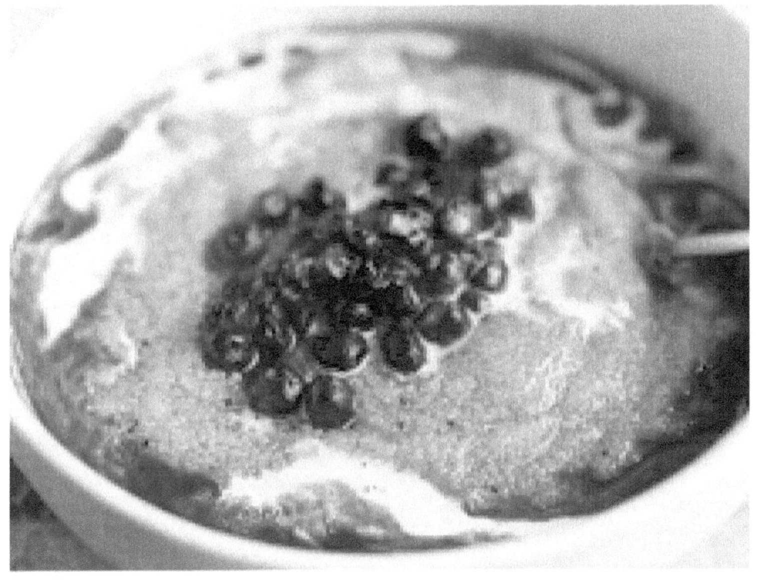

Preparation Time: 10 minutes

Cook Time: 30 minutes

Serves: 2 servings

Ingredients

2 cup filtered water

1/3 cup whole-grain amaranth

1 tablespoon maple syrup

¼ cup hemp seeds

½ cup blueberries

1 teaspoon cinnamon

1 (chopped) medium pear

Instructions

1. Add water and the amaranth into a well lidded nonstick cast iron skillet over med-heat.

2. Bring mixture to boiling.

3. Place lid over skillet and adjust heat to low.

4. Simmer amaranth until liquid evaporates, for 25-30 minutes.

TIP: To prevent sticking, stir amaranth once every 10 minutes.

5. Take skillet off heat and stir cinnamon, maple syrup and hemp seeds into the skillet mixture until combined.

6. Split cereal into 2 serving bowls, topped with pear and blueberries.

Cherry Coconut Porridge

Preparation Time: 5 minutes

Cook Time: 20 minutes

Serves: 5 servings

Ingredients

4 tbsps chia seed

1 1/2 cups oats

3 tbsps raw cacao

3-4 cups reduced fat coconut milk

5 tablespoons coconut shavings

1 pinch of stevia

5 teaspoons dark chocolate shavings

1/2 cup (pitted) frozen or fresh cherries

2 tablespoons maple syrup

Instructions

1. Add stevia, cacao, coconut milk, chia and oats into a saucepan over med-heat.

2. Combine mixture and bring to boiling.

3. Adjust heat to med-low and simmer until the oats are well cooked.

4. Pour oats into serving bowls, topped with maple syrup, dark chocolate shavings, cherries, and coconut shavings.

5. Enjoy.

Ginger Buckwheat Granola

Preparation Time: 15 minutes

Cook Time: 50 minutes

Serves: 1 big bowl

Ingredients

1 cup buckwheat

2 cups oats

1 cup pumpkin seeds

1 cup sunflower seeds

1 cup apple puree

1 ½ cups dates, pitted

4 tbsps raw cacao powder

6 tbsps coconut oil

1 piece of ginger, peeled & grated

Instructions

1. Heat up oven to 350°F.

2. Add seeds, buckwheat and oats into a big mixing bowl and stir until well combined.

3. Add apple puree, coconut oil and dates into a saucepan over med-low heat.

4. Simmer until dates are tender and nice, for 5 minutes.

5. Add grated ginger into the date mixture and stir until incorporated.

6. Add the date mixture into a high speed electric blender.

7. Add raw cacao powder into the blender also and process until a fine and smooth consistency is reached.

8. Pour the blended date mixture over oats bowl and stir until well combined and coated.

9. Prepare a big coconut oil greased baking tray.

10. Spread granola over pregreased baking tray and transfer baking tray into the preheated oven.

11. Bake until crispy and nice, for about 45 minutes.

NOTE: Take out baking tray at the 15-minute cook time mark, and stir granola until combined to prevent burning, and repeat stirring every 5-10 minutes while cooking.

12. Remove granola from the oven and let sit until cooled.

13. Store granola into a well lidded container, for about 30 days.

Almond-Berry Smoothie Bowl

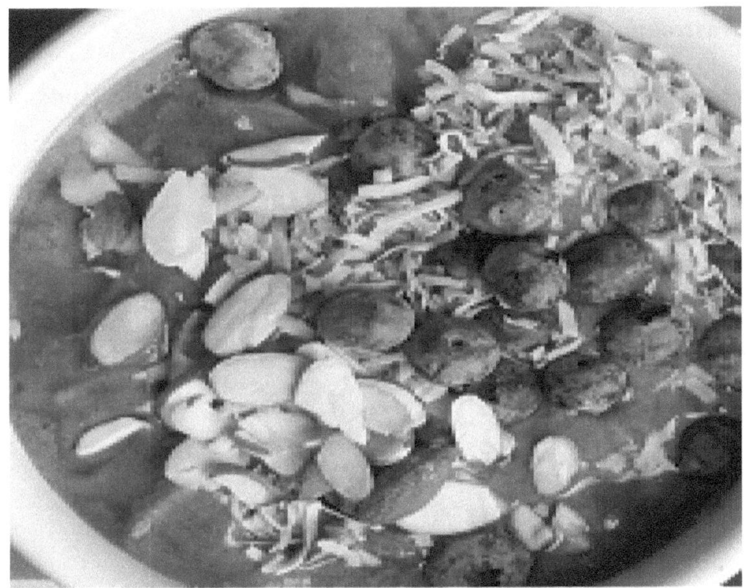

Preparation Time: 10 minutes

Cook Time: 0 minutes

Serves: 1 serving

Ingredients

½ cup sliced banana, frozen

1/3 cup raspberries, frozen

5 tbsps (divided) almonds, sliced

½ cup almond milk, plain unsweetened

1/3 tsp cardamom, ground

¼ tsp cinnamon, ground

¼ cup raspberries

1/3 tsp vanilla extract

1 tbsp coconut flakes, unsweetened

Instructions

1. Add vanilla, cardamom, cinnamon, 3 tbsps almonds, almond milk, banana and raspberries into a high speed electric blender.

2. Blend mixture until a smooth consistency is reached.

3. Transfer blended smoothie mixture into a bowl, topped with the coconut, the remaining almonds and the raspberries.

4. Serve and enjoy.

Spinach Mushroom Frittata

Preparation Time: 15 minutes

Cook Time: 30 minutes

Serves: 4 servings

Ingredients

1/4 cup milk

6 eggs

1 (sliced thin) onion

1 cup cheddar cheese, grated

3 tbsps butter

4 ounces (sliced) white button mushrooms

Salt and pepper

2 cups baby spinach

Instructions

1. Heat up oven to 350°F and set the rack in the center position.

2. Coat an 8" square baking dish with butter and let sit.

3. Add milk and eggs into a big bowl and whisk until combined.

4. Sprinkle pepper and salt over the egg mixture and set egg bowl aside.

5. Add mushrooms and onions into a big skillet over med-heat and brown.

6. Season with pepper and salt.

7. Add spinach into the skillet and stir cook continuously, for about 1 minute.

8. Add mushroom mixture into the egg bowl and stir until well combined.

9. Pour mushroom egg mixture into the prepared baking sheet.

10. Place baking sheet in the preheated oven and bake until puffed and lightly browned, for about 25 minutes.

11. Slice frittata into 4 squares and take out from baking dish using a spatula.

12. Serve and enjoy.

Delicious Crepes

Preparation Time: 10 minutes

Cook Time: 10 minutes

Serves: 6 servings

Ingredients

1 tsp gluten-free vanilla

2 eggs

1/2 cup water

1/2 cup nut milk

1-2 tbsps agave nectar

1/4 tsp salt

2 tbsps melted coconut oil

1 cup all purpose flour, gluten-free

1 tbsps coconut oil

Instructions

1. Melt 2 tbsps coconut oil into a small saucepan over low-heat.

2. Add agave nectar, salt, water, nut milk, vanilla and eggs into a fairly big bowl and whisk until combined.

3. Add in the flour into the bowl and slowly whisk until combined.

4. Pour melted coconut oil in a slow and steady stream and continuously whisk until combined.

5. Stir mixture until a smooth consistency is reached.

6. Add a little amount of coconut oil into a big frying pan over med-high heat.

7. Scoop batter 1/3 cup of batter per crepe onto the griddle.

8. Swirl and tilt pan in a round motion until batter evenly covers griddle surface.

9. Cook until crepes bottom is light brown, for about 2 minutes.

10. Using a spatula, flip crepe and cook other side.

11. Serve and enjoy

Delicious Morning Toast

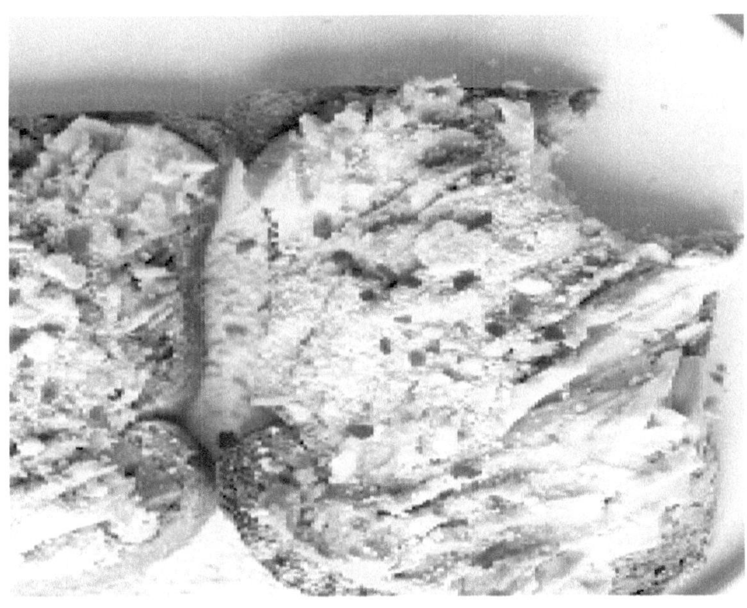

Preparation Time: 5 minutes

Cook Time: 0 minutes

Serves: 1 serving

Ingredients

1 lime, juiced

2 whole grain bread slices

Olive oil

1 avocado

Chili flakes

Instructions

1. Drizzle olive oil over toast bread slices.

2. Drizzle with lime juice.

3. Top toast bread slices with avocado slices and sprinkle with chili flakes.

4. Cover sandwich with the other toast slice.

5. Serve and enjoy.

Raspberry Almond Butter Smoothie

Preparation Time: 5 minutes

Cook Time: 0 minutes

Serves: 1 serving

Ingredients

1/2 ripe banana, medium

1/4 cup 1% low-fat milk

1 cup fresh raspberries or frozen

1 tablespoon creamy almond butter

1/2 cup crushed ice

Instructions

1. Add every ingredient into a high speed electric blender.

2. Blend until a creamy and smooth consistency is reached.

Peach Matcha Smoothie Bowl

Preparation Time: 10 minutes

Cook Time: 0 minutes

Serves: 1 serving

Ingredients

¾ cup coconut milk, unsweetened

1 cup sliced peaches, frozen

¼ cup silken tofu

½ cup avocado, diced

1 tsp matcha tea powder

2 tsps honey

1 tbsp almonds, roughly chopped

¼ cup fresh blackberries

1 tsp hemp seeds

1 tbsp coconut flakes, unsweetened

Instructions

1. Add matcha, honey, tofu, avocado, coconut milk and peaches into a high speed electric blender.

2. Blend mixture until a smooth consistency is reached.

3. Transfer blended smoothie into a bowl, topped with hemp seeds, coconut flakes, almonds and blackberries.

4. Serve and enjoy.

Turmeric Chia Pudding

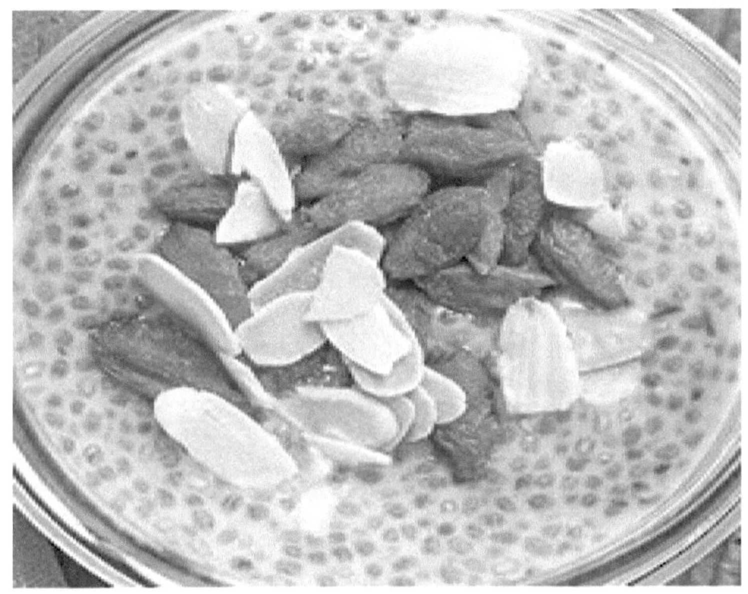

Preparation Time: 3 minutes

Cook Time: 0 minutes

Serves: 2-4 servings

Ingredients

1/3 cup chia seeds

1 1/2 cups almond milk

1 teaspoon turmeric, ground

2 tablespoons honey

1/8 teaspoon cardamom, ground

1/2 teaspoon cinnamon

1/8 teaspoon cloves, ground

Instructions

1. Add every ingredient into a bowl.

2. Pour into jars and let sit over the night.

3. Serve, topped with berries and nuts.

Berry Yogurt Parfait

Preparation Time: 5 minutes

Cook Time: 0 minutes

Serves: 1 serving

Ingredients

1/2 cup strawberries, sliced

1 cup Greek yogurt, nonfat plain

2 tablespoons nonfat granola

1/2 banana

Stevia drops

Instructions

1. Add yogurt and stevia into a bowl and mix until combined.

2. Arrange bananas, yogurt mixture and strawberries alternately into a glass until filled.

3. Top parfait with a generous sprinkle of granola and place in a refrigerator until chilled.

4. Serve parfait and enjoy.

Poached Eggs with Curried Potatoes

Preparation Time: 10 minutes

Cook Time: 30 minutes

Serves: 4 servings

Ingredients

1" fresh ginger

2 (about 2 pounds) russet potatoes, washed & cut into 3/4" cubes

1 tablespoon extra-virgin olive oil

2 (peeled and minced) garlic cloves

15 ounce can tomato sauce

2 tablespoons (hot or mild) curry powder

1/2 bunch fresh cilantro, if desired

4 big eggs

Instructions

1. Add just enough water to cover and the potato cubes into a big pot over high heat.

2. Place lid over pot and bring mixture to boiling.

3. Boil potato cubes until softened, for 5-6 minutes.

4. Pour the cooked potato cubes in a colander and drain.

5. Add olive oil into a big deep skillet over med-low heat.

6. Add garlic and ginger into the oil and saute until aromatic and tender, for 1-2 minutes.

7. Add curry powder into the skillet and saute until toasted for 1 minute.

8. Stir in tomato sauce into the skillet until combined.

9. Adjust heat to med-heat.

10. Cook sauce until heated through.

11. Check for seasoning and adjust salt if desired.

12. Add the drained potato cubes into the skillet and stir until covered with sauce.

TIP: if potato mixture seems too pasty or dry, add few tbsps water.

13. Make 4 wells in the potato mixture.

14. Add one cracked egg into each well, until all wells are filled with egg.

15. Cover skillet and simmer potato egg mixture.

16. Simmer mixture until egg is cooked through, for 6-10 minutes.

17. Top poached eggs and curried potatoes with chopped fresh cilantro.

18. Serve and enjoy.

Apple Ginger Rhubarb Muffins

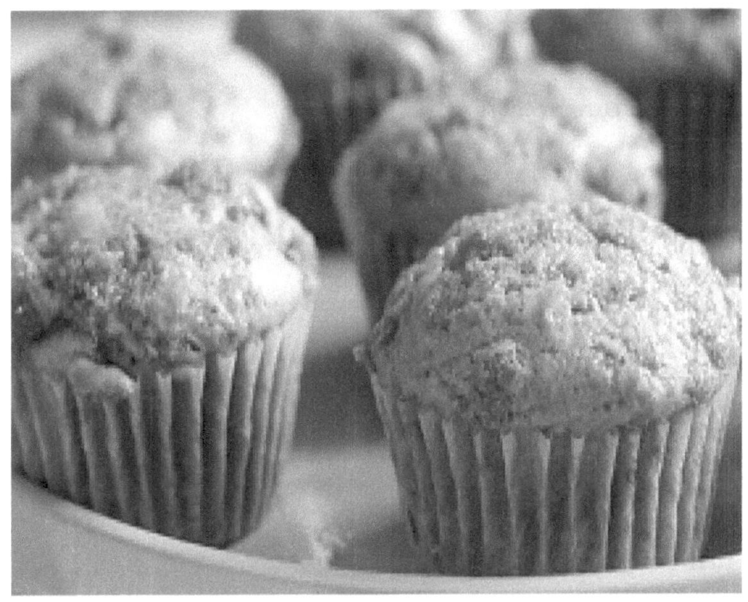

Preparation Time: 10 minutes

Cook Time: 25 minutes

Serves: 8 servings

Ingredients

1/4 cup unrefined raw sugar

1/2 cup almond meal

1 tbsp linseed meal, ground

2 tbsps crystallized ginger, finely chopped

1/4 cup fine brown rice flour

1/2 cup buckwheat flour

2 tsps baking powder, gluten-free

2 tbsps organic cornflour

1/2 tsp ginger, ground

1/2 tsp cinnamon, ground

1 cup rhubarb, finely sliced

1 generous pinch fine sea salt

1/3 cup almond milk plus 1 tbsp

1 (peeled, cored and diced finely) small apple

1 large egg, organic

1/4 cup extra-virgin olive oil

1 tsp vanilla extract

Instructions

1. Heat up oven to 350°F.

2. Prepare 8 paper cases lined muffin tins.

TIP: Each muffin tin should be having a 1/3 cup capacity.

3. Add linseed meal, ginger, sugar and almond meal into a fairly big bowl.

4. Sift flours, spices and baking powder.

5. Whisk flour mixture until well combined.

6. Add apple and rhubarb into the flour mixture and stir until wholly coated.

7. Add vanilla, egg, oil and milk into a separate bowl and whisk until combined.

8. Pour wet mixture into the dry mixture and stir until combined.

9. Split batter into prepared muffin tins and transfer into the preheated oven.

10. Bake muffins until golden around the edges and muffin is raised, for 20-25 minutes.

TIP: Check for doneness, by inserting a toothpick in the middle of a muffin and see if it comes out clean.

11. Take muffin tin out of the oven and let sit until slightly cooled for 5 minutes.

12. Transfer to a wire rack until wholly cooled.

13. Serve and eat warm or keep in a well lidded container for 2-3 days.

Lunch Recipes

Buckwheat Pasta with Roasted Red Pepper and Tomato

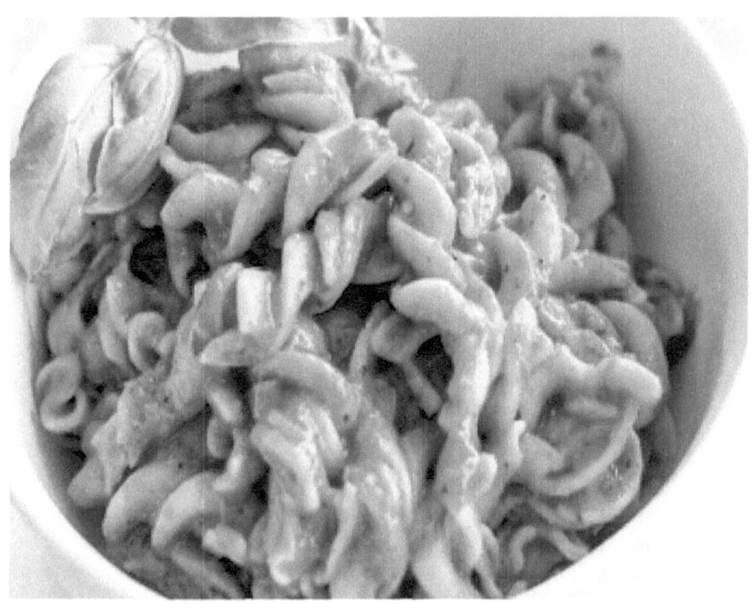

Preparation Time: 10 minutes

Cook Time: 20 minutes

Serves: 2 servings

Ingredients

10-12 (rinsed, cleaned & chopped) tomatoes

4 large (cored & chopped) red peppers

3 (peeled & chopped) garlic cloves

6-8 fresh basil leaves

2 tbsps olive oil

2 (chopped) spring onion stalks

Dried mixed herbs, as necessary

1 tsp rice malt syrup

2 cups buckwheat pasta

Salt and pepper, as necessary

Instructions

1. Heat up oven to 350°F.

2. Prepare a parchment paper lined baking tray.

3. Spread the red peppers and tomatoes on the prepared baking tray.

4. Season tomato mixture with mixed dried herbs, pepper and salt to taste.

5. Place baking tray into the preheated oven and roast for 10 minutes.

6. Add spring onion and chopped garlic into the tray, drizzled with olive oil and return baking tray into the preheated oven.

7. Roast mixture for 10 more minutes.

8. In the meantime, add water into a pot over med-high heat.

9. Bring to boiling; add 1 pinch of salt with the buckwheat pasta.

10. Cook pasta according to package directions.

11. Take out veggies from the oven and let sit until cool.

12. Add the cooled roasted veggies into a high speed electric blender.

13. Blend until a creamy and smooth sauce consistency is reached.

14. Add rice malt syrup into the blender and blend until incorporated.

15. Drain pasta and rinse quickly under cold water to stop cooking.

16. Return tomato sauce and pasta into the pot and stir until combined.

17. Heat pasta gently until warmed through.

18. Serve garnished with pepper, salt, nutritional yeast and fresh basil.

Chickpea Cakes with Turmeric

Preparation Time: 5 minutes

Cook Time: 10 minutes

Serves: 4 servings

Ingredients

2 garlic cloves

1 small onion

1 small bunch (coarsely chopped) fresh parsley

1 can chickpeas, rinsed & drained

1-2 tsps sea salt

2 tbsps potato starch

1 tsp turmeric powder

Freshly ground black pepper

5 tbsps (divided) chickpea flour

1/2–1 tsp cayenne pepper, if desired

Olive oil

Instructions

1. Add olive oil into a big cast iron pan over med-heat.

2. Add garlic and onion into the hot oil and saute until just golden.

NOTE: Do not burn.

3. Take off pan and let sit until cooled.

4. Add chickpeas into a food processor and blend until a slightly paste-like consistency is reached

5. Add cayenne pepper, turmeric, pepper, salt, garlic and onion into the food processor and pulse until combined.

6. Add chopped parsley and stir until combined.

7. Sprinkle about 2-3 tbsps chickpea flour on a big plate.

8. Scoop batter from the food processor and shape into ball-like patties.

TIP: Each patty should about the size of a golf ball.

9. Drop each patty into the chickpea flour into evenly coated.

NOTE: Gently dust off excess flour.

10. Place the same pan you used over med-heat.

11. Add olive oil into the pan and cook until nicely browned on each side, for about 2-3 minutes per side.

12. Serve with salad or vegetables and enjoy.

Freekeh Meatballs

Preparation Time: 15 minutes

Cook Time: 50 minutes

Serves: 8 servings

Ingredients

2 1/2 cups water

1 cup cracked freekeh, uncooked

1 (grated) medium onion

1 (grated) small potato

1/2 cup finely chopped parsley

2 minced garlic cloves

3/4 cup grated Pecorino Romano cheese

3/4 cup bread crumbs

1/4 teaspoon black pepper, freshly ground

3 (whisked) eggs

2 tablespoons olive oil

1/2 teaspoon salt

Instructions

1. Add freekeh and water into a big saucepan over med-heat.

2. Bring mixture to boiling.

3. Stir and adjust heat to simmering.

4. Stir again and place lid over saucepan.

5. Cook freekeh for 20 minutes, remove and let cool.

6. Drain and add every other ingredient excluding the olive oil into the bowl with the cooled freekeh.

7. Mix freekeh mixture until combined.

8. Place freekeh mixture in a refrigerator for 1 hour or more.

9. Heat up oven to 400°F.

10. Prepare 2 parchment paper lined cookie sheets.

11. Coat each parchment paper lined cookie sheet with 1 tbsp olive oil.

12. Make 26 meatballs from the freekeh mixture, using clean hands and making sure you do not press balls.

13. Arrange 13 meatballs on each prepared cookie sheet.

14. Place cookie sheets in the preheated oven and bake until deeply golden, for 20 minutes.

15. Flip meatballs with an oven-safe spatula and bake until golden, for 5-10 more minutes.

16. Serve meatballs and enjoy.

Baked Apples Stuffed with Seeds, Nuts and Cinnamon

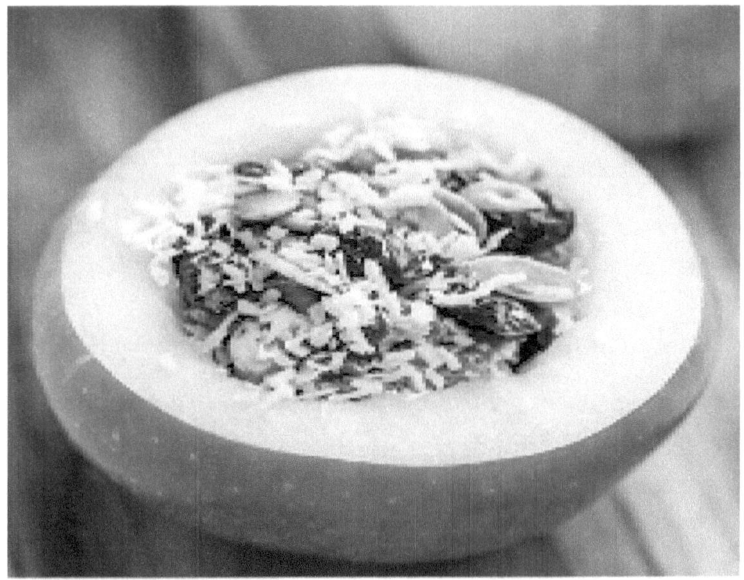

Preparation Time: 5 minutes

Cook Time: 35 minutes

Serves: 4 servings

Ingredients

¼ cup cranberries, dried

½ cups seeds & nuts mix (walnuts, almonds, cashews, hemp seeds, and flax seeds)

1 teaspoon fresh ginger root, grated

2 (pitted & chopped) dates

½ teaspoon nutmeg

1 teaspoon cinnamon

4 apples, (skin-on, cut out core without cutting through the bottom)

¼ teaspoon cloves, ground

1 cup lemon juice

¼ cup liquid honey, unpasteurized

Instructions

1. Heat up oven to 325°F.

2. Add spices, ginger root, dates, cranberries and seeds/nuts mixture into a bowl and combine.

3. Add the seed/nut mixture into the hole made in each apple until filled.

4. Dribble honey over stuffing and transfer stuffed apple onto an 8-by-8" baking dish.

5. Pour lemon juice around the apples in the baking dish to moisten.

6. Transfer baking dish into the preheated oven and bake until apples are tender, for 30-35 minutes.

7. Serve warm.

Vegetable Burger with Quinoa and Beet

Preparation Time: 10 minutes

Cook Time: 10 minutes

Serves: 8 servings

Ingredients (Burger)

5 tbsps (divided) flax meal

1 1/2 cups eggplant, chopped

4 cups beets, shredded

6 tbsps warm water

1 cup rolled oats, gluten-free

1 cup quinoa, cooked

1/2 cup hummus

2 minced garlic cloves

Salt and pepper, to taste

Serve with

Greens

Gluten-free buns

Hummus

Instructions

1. Add chopped eggplant into a steaming basket.

2. Steam the chopped eggplants for about 5 minutes, until are fork tender.

3. Place tenderized eggplants into a food processor or high speed electric blender.

4. Blend on high until a smooth consistency is reached.

5. Pour blended eggplants into a bowl and let sit until needed.

6. Add water and 2 tbsps flaxmeal into a small bowl and stir quickly.

7. Add garlic, the remaining 3 tbsps flaxmeal, oats, quinoa and beets into a food processor.

8. Process mixture until combine and pour into a big bowl.

9. Add the water and flax mixture with the hummus and blended eggplants into the oats-quinoa bowl.

10. Mix batter until the dough firms up and can be shaped into patties.

11. Season dough with pepper and salt.

NOTE: If dough is too moist, set dough aside for 10-15 minutes before adding more water and flax mixture into the dough.

12. Prepare a parchment paper lined baking sheet.

13. Using clean hands, shape dough into 8 patties.

14. Place shaped patties onto the prepared baking sheet and refrigerate for 60 minutes or more until chilled.

15. Add a little amount of oil into a big skillet over med-heat.

16. Add burgers into the hot oil, working in batches, and sear for about 3-4 minutes on each side.

17. Place cooked burgers on a wire rack.

18. Repeat process until all burgers is well cooked.

19. Serve burgers with the gluten-free buns, topped with a smear of hummus and the greens.

Tomato Salsa with Sweet Potato Frittata

Preparation Time: 10 minutes

Cook Time: 10 minutes

Serves: 2 servings

Ingredients (Frittata)

1 tbsp olive oil

1 (7-8 ounces) big sweet potato {peel & slice into 1/2" cubes)

Sea salt

1 (peeled & minced) shallot

4 big eggs

Black pepper

1 small handful (finely sniped) chives

Tomato Salsa

2 (trimmed & sliced thin diagonally) green onions

8 oz. vine-ripened plum tomatoes, sliced into halves

1/2 lime, juiced

1 handful (chopped) cilantro leaves

1 tbsp sesame oil

3 tbsps olive oil

1-2 drops honey, to taste (if desired)

1 dash Tabasco sauce

Instructions

1. Add tomato halves into a big bowl.

2. Add every other salsa ingredient into the big bowl and mix until combined.

3. Season with pepper and salt as necessary and honey, if desired.

4. Let salsa sit until needed.

5. Preheat broiler to the highest temperature.

6. Add olive oil into an oven-secure skillet over med-heat.

7. Add shallot and potato into the skillet and sprinkle liberally with pepper and salt.

8. Cook until potato edges are lightly golden and potatoes are just softened, for about 4-5 minutes.

9. Crack eggs into a bowl and beat.

10. Add chives into the egg and whisk to combine.

11. Add the eggs and chives mixture into the skillet over the sweet potatoes.

12. Shake pan until the mixture is evenly combined and distributed.

13. Adjust heat to low-heat, and cook until eggs set at the edges and bottom, for some minutes.

TIP: Do not stir.

14. Place skillet under the preheated broiler and broil until the frittata sets.

15. Set aside for 1 minute.

16. Remove frittata from skillet and flip onto a big plate.

17. Scoop tomato salsa over frittata, serve at once and enjoy.

Roasted Chickpeas with Turmeric

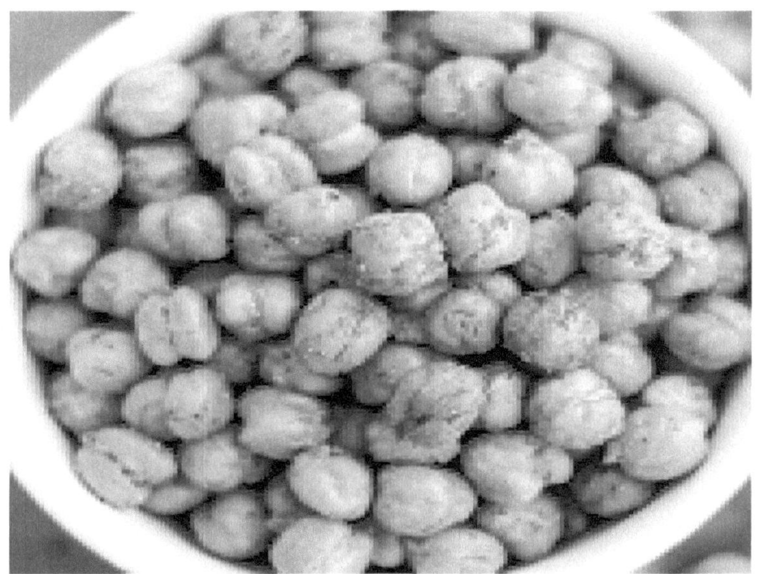

Preparation Time: 10 minutes

Cook Time: 40 minutes

Serves: 1 (15 oz.) serving

Ingredients

1/2 tsp paprika

1 tsp turmeric

1 tsp salt

1/4 tsp black pepper

1 can (rinsed) chickpeas

2 tsp olive oil

Instructions

1. Toss chickpeas with spices, salt and olive oil on a parchment paper lined baking sheet.

2. Transfer baking sheet into an oven preheated to 425°F.

3. Roast chickpeas for 30 minutes, stirring twice while roasting.

4. Place roasted chickpeas in a well lidded container at room temperature.

5. Serve and enjoy.

Turmeric Quinoa Bowls

Preparation Time: 30 minutes

Cook Time: 30 minutes

Serves: 4 servings

Ingredients

1 (15 ounces) can chickpeas, drained & rinsed

7 (sliced into strips) small yellow potatoes

1 teaspoon paprika

2 teaspoons turmeric

1/4 cup quinoa

1 tablespoon coconut oil

Freshly ground black pepper

Sea salt

1/2 tablespoon olive oil

2 (washed) kale leaves

1 (peeled, pitted and sliced) avocado

Instructions

1. Heat up oven to 350°F.

2. Lay potato strips on one-half of a baking sheet, sprinkle with 1 teaspoon turmeric and drizzle with coconut oil.

3. Season potato strips with pepper and salt as desired.

4. Place baking sheet into the preheated oven and roast for 5 minutes.

5. Add 1 teaspoon paprika and chickpeas into a bowl and mix until wholly coated.

6. Transfer chickpeas into the empty side of the baking sheet.

7. Return into the oven and roast potatoes and chickpeas until the potatoes are tenderized, for about 25 minutes.

8. Add 1/2 cup of water and quinoa into a pot over med-high heat.

9. Cook quinoa until well cooked.

10. Add pepper, salt to taste and 1 teaspoon turmeric into the quinoa and stir until combined.

11. Let quinoa sit until cooled.

12. Rub olive oil over washed kale leaves and split kale leaves into 4 serving bowls.

13. Split avocado slices into the bowls and top with the roasted potatoes, chickpeas and quinoa.

Spicy Veggie Burgers with Cilantro Avocado Crema

Preparation Time: 55 minutes

Cook Time: 10 minutes

Serves: 6 servings

Ingredients

1 can (rinsed & drained) black beans

1/2 cup quinoa, rinsed with cold water

1/2 cup red onion, diced

1 sweet potato, large

1/2 cup cilantro, chopped

2 minced garlic cloves

1 tsp cumin

1/2 (seeded & diced) jalapeno

1/4 oat bran, gluten free

2 tsps cajun seasoning, spicy

Extra-virgin olive oil

Salt and pepper, as desired

Sprouts

6 whole grain hamburger buns

Cilantro Avocado Crema

1/4 cup plain Greek yogurt

1/2 (diced) big ripe avocado

1 tsp lemon juice

2 tbsps cilantro, chopped

Salt, as necessary

1 dash of hot sauce

Instructions

1. Add 1 cup of water into a fairly big saucepan.

2. Bring water to boiling.

3. Add quinoa into the hot water and bring to boiling.

4. Place lid over saucepan and adjust heat to low heat.

5. Keep simmering quinoa until liquid is fully absorbed, for 15 minutes.

6. Take off heat and using a fork, fluff quinoa.

7. Add quinoa into a big bowl and let sit for about 10 minutes until cooled.

8. Use a fork to pierce sweet potato in several places and transfer into a microwave.

9. Heat sweet potatoes until well cooked and tender, for about 3-4 minutes.

NOTE: Don't overcook.

10. Peel potato skin once cooled.

11. Add Cajun seasoning, cumin, garlic, cilantro, red onion, cooked sweet potato and beans into a food processor.

12. Pulse mixture until a smooth consistency is reached.

13. Pour beans mixture into the quinoa bowl and mix until combined.

14. Season with pepper and salt as needed.

15. Add about 1/3 cup oat bran into the quinoa mixture and mix until combined and shape into patties.

16. Form batter into 6 even patties and transfer onto a baking sheet lined with parchment paper.

17. Transfer patties into a refrigerator for 30 minutes or more.

18. Add lemon juice, cilantro, diced avocado and yogurt into a food processor and blend until a smooth consistency is reached.

19. Season with salt, as necessary

20. Place crema in a refrigerator until needed.

21. Place a skillet over med-high heat.

22. Add olive oil into the hot skillet.

23. Place patties in the hot oil and fry until golden brown, for about 3-4 minutes on each side.

24. Serve patties with desired toppings, crema, sprouts and hamburger buns.

Dinner Recipes

Spaghetti Squash Stuffed with Chickpea and Kale

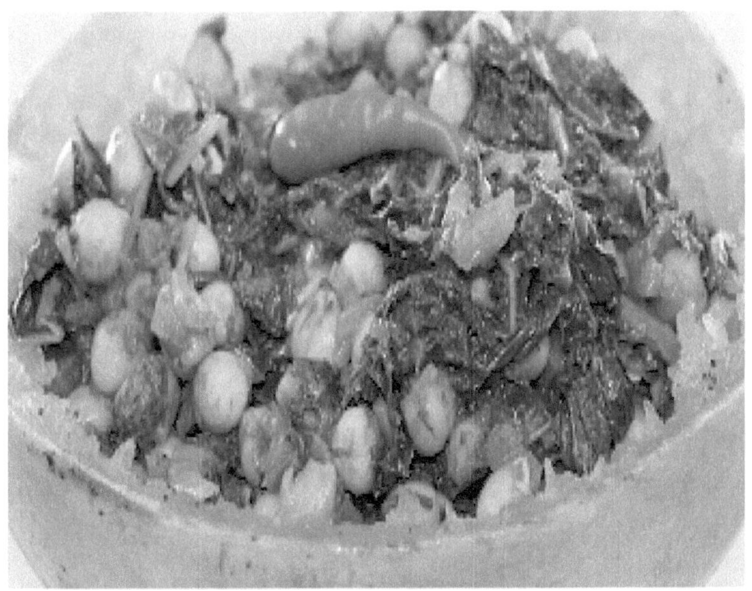

Preparation Time: 10 minutes

Cook Time: 40 minutes

Serves: 2 servings

Ingredients

4-5 handfuls (washed & big stems removed) kale

1 (halved, seeded and stringed) spaghetti squash

1 cup (drained & rinsed) chickpeas

2 minced garlic cloves

Olive oil

1/4 cup almonds, slivered

Sea salt and pepper

Instructions

1. Heat up oven to 400°F.

2. Lightly brush each squash half inside with olive oil and season with pepper and sea salt.

3. Transfer squash halves onto a baking sheet with the hollow side down.

4. Place baking sheet into the preheated oven and bake for 40 minutes.

5. In the meantime, add olive oil into a fairly big skillet over med-heat.

6. Add the minced garlic into the hot oil and saute for 1 minute.

7. Add the slivered almonds into the skillet with the garlic and cook for some more minutes, until the almonds are just beginning to toast and garlic is aromatic.

8. Add kale into the skillet mixture and season with salt.

9. Saute kale mixture, stirring until combined and wilted.

10. Add chickpea into the skillet mixture and stir until combined.

11. Split kale mixture between squash halves.

12. Serve and enjoy.

Kale, Tomato, Chickpeas with Braised Cauliflower

Preparation Time: 10 minutes

Cook Time: 1 hour 15 minutes

Serves: 3-4 servings

Ingredients

1 big (leaves & stems removed) whole cauliflower

2 tbsps olive oil

1 (15 oz.) can {drained & rinsed} chickpeas

1 (28 oz.) can tomato, crushed

1/4 cup nutritional yeast, if desired

5-6 kale leaves

2 tsps oregano, dried

3 minced garlic cloves

Salt and pepper, as necessary

Instructions

1. Heat up oven to 350°F.

2. Add oil into a Dutch oven over med-high heat.

3. Add cauliflower into the hot oil and sear for about 10 minutes, until the cauliflower outside is brown.

TIP: Continue to rotate cauliflower while cooking.

4. Take out the cauliflower and place on a cutting board.

5. Add pepper, salt, oregano, garlic, nutritional yeast, kale, chickpeas and tomato into the Dutch oven and cook for 3-4 more minutes.

6. Add cauliflower into the tomato mixture in the pot and coat cauliflower evenly.

7. Transfer Dutch oven into an oven and bake for about 1 hour, until softened.

8. Take out braised cauliflower from the oven and let sit until cooled before slicing.

9. Serve sliced cauliflower, topped with a generous scoop of the tomato mixture.

Avocado Dipping Sauce with Roasted Sweet Potatoes

Preparation Time: 10 minutes

Cook Time: 45 minutes

Serves: 4 servings

Ingredients

1 tsp olive oil

2 (washed & sliced into 1/2" cubes) big sweet potatoes

1 (halved) avocado

1/2 tsp sea salt

1 lemon, juiced

1 (peeled & chopped) big garlic clove

2 tbsp olive oil

2-4 tbsp water

Instructions

1. Heat up oven to 400°F.

2. Place sweet potato cubes on a baking pan and spread in one layer.

3. Drizzle sweet potato cubes with olive oil.

4. Use clean hands to turn potatoes over until completely and lightly covered with olive oil.

5. Season potatoes with 1/4 tsp salt and transfer baking pan into the preheated oven.

6. Bake sweet potatoes until potato tops are lightly browned, for 40-45 minutes.

7. Add potato flesh into a high speed electric blender.

8. Add 1/4 tsp salt, lemon juice and garlic into the blender.

9. Blend avocado mixture until a smooth and creamy consistency is reached.

10. Add little water into the mixture and blend until very smooth.

11. Dribble in olive oil in a slow and steady stream while blending until a creamy and smooth consistency is reached.

12. Serve roasted potatoes with dipping sauce and enjoy.

Squash Red Lentil Curry Stew

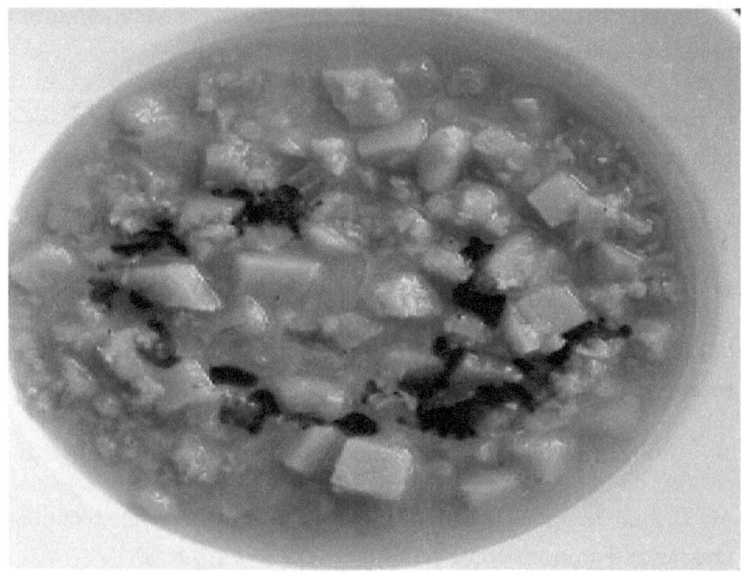

Preparation Time: 10 minutes

Cook Time: 30 minutes

Serves: 4 servings

Ingredients

1 chopped sweet onion

1 teaspoon extra-virgin olive oil

1 tablespoon curry powder

3 minced garlic cloves

1 cup red lentils

4 cups low-sodium broth

1 cup greens of choice

3 cups butternut squash, cooked

1/2 teaspoon kosher salt and black pepper

Fresh grated ginger, if desired

Instructions

1. Add olive oil into a big pot over med-low heat.

2. Add minced garlic and chopped onion into the oil and saute for about 5 minutes.

3. Add curry powder into the mixture, stir until combined and cook for some minutes.

4. Add lentils and broth into the mixture and bring to boiling.

5. Lower heat and cook for 10 more minutes.

6. Add cooked butternut into the pot and stir until incorporated.

7. Cook for about 5-8 minutes over med-heat.

8. Sprinkle freshly grated ginger, pepper and salt over mixture.

9. Serve and enjoy.

Broccolini and Quinoa with Sesame-Orange Salmon

Preparation Time: 10 minutes

Cook Time: 15 minutes

Serves: 4 servings

Ingredients

½ cup (divided) orange juice + 1/3 cup

1 cup quinoa

1 (trimmed) bunch broccolini

2 sliced scallions

½ tsp (divided) ground pepper

1 tbsp extra-virgin olive oil

¼ tsp garlic powder

3 tsps (divided) sesame oil, toasted

1 tsp black sesame seeds

4 (4-oz.) portions wild salmon

1 tbsp tamari, reduced-sodium

1 tbsp fresh ginger, minced

1 tsp cornstarch

Instructions

1. Cook quinoa according to instructions on the package.

NOTE: Substitute 1/2 cup orange for 1/2 cup water.

2. Take off cooked quinoa from heat and add scallions.

3. Stir until incorporated, place lid over pot and let sit until needed.

4. Heat up oven to 450°F.

5. Prepare a rimmed aluminum foil lined baking sheet.

6. Add broccolini into a big bowl and toss with 1/4 tsp pepper, 1/4 tsp salt and oil.

7. Lay seasoned broccolini onto the baking sheet and transfer baking sheet into the preheated oven.

8. Roast broccolini for 8 minutes.

9. In the meantime, add 1/4 tsp pepper, 1/4 tsp salt, garlic powder and 2 tsp sesame oil into a small bowl and stir until combined.

10. Brush salmon with the pepper and oil mixture.

11. Add salmon to a side of the baking pan, pushing roasted broccolini to the opposite side.

12. Bake salmon for 5-8 minutes until cooked through.

13. Sprinkle sesame seeds over salmon.

14. Add cornstarch, tamari, ginger, 1 tsp sesame oil and 1/3 cup orange juice into a small oven-secure bowl and whisk until combined.

15. Place bowl in a microwave and heat for 1 minute on high.

16. Split salmon, broccolini and quinoa between four plates.

17. Drizzle 2 tbsps sauce over each plate.

18. Serve and enjoy.

Vegetarian Chili

Preparation Time: 15 minutes

Cook Time: 1 hour 40 minutes

Serves: 4 servings

Ingredients

1 cup onions

2 tablespoons olive oil

1 red pepper

1 poblano pepper

1 small sweet potato

2 mushrooms

2 tablespoons cumin, ground

2 garlic cloves

2 chili peppers

1 tablespoon oregano, dried

28 ounces diced tomatoes

2 small dried red chilies

16 ounces corn kernels, frozen

15 ounces low sodium beans

2 tablespoons basil, dried

2 tablespoons oregano, dried

2 bay leaves

1 tablespoon chili powder

Vegetable broth

Instructions

1. Add sweet potatoes, mushrooms, red pepper, poblano pepper and onions into a big Dutch oven over med-heat.

2. Saute for about 7 minutes until veggies are tender.

3. Add the red chilies and chili pepper into the pot and stir until incorporated.

4. Cook for 1 more minute.

5. Add the bay leaves, chili powder, basil, oregano, corn, beans and tomatoes into the pot and add some vegetable broth as needed.

6. Cook chili for about 1 hour 30 minutes on low.

7. Get rid of the bay leaves.

8. Serve chili into bowls, top each bowl with a lemon wedge, sour cream and a little amount of shredded cheese.

Turkey White Bean Chili Blanco

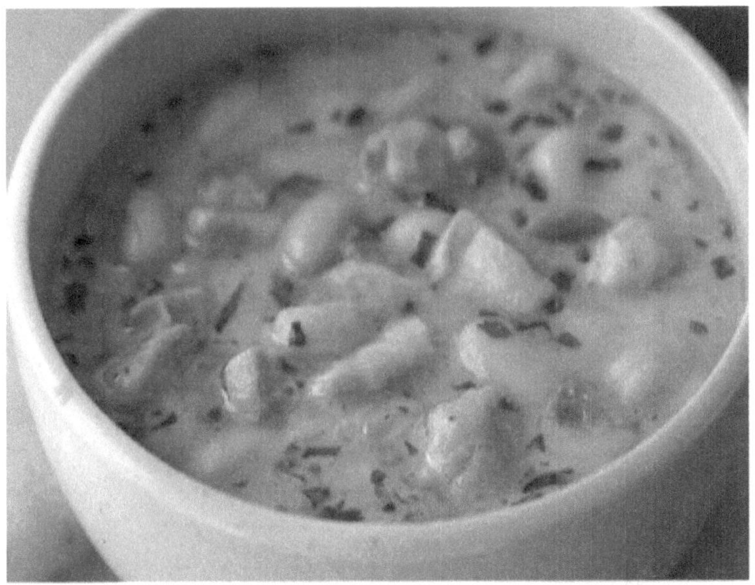

Preparation Time: 20 minutes

Cook Time: 1 hour

Serves: 8-10 servings

Ingredients

2 tbsps olive oil

1 lb. (chopped into small chunks) turkey breasts, boneless & skinless

2 garlic cloves

1 diced medium onion

1 cup (frozen & thawed or fresh) corn kernels

2 (15-oz.) cans (drained & rinsed) white beans

2 tsps cumin, ground

1 (4-oz.) can green chiles, chopped

1/8 tsp cayenne pepper

2 tsps pure chili powder

2 cups Monterey Jack cheese, grated

3 cups water

2 tbsps fresh chopped cilantro

Instructions

1. Sprinkle pepper and salt over turkey until well seasoned.

2. Add oil into a big saucepan over high heat.

3. Add turkey pieces into the hot oil and stir cook for 2-3 minutes until browned.

4. Adjust heat to med-heat.

5. Add garlic and onion into the turkey mixture and cook for 5-6 minutes until the onion becomes translucent.

6. Add water, spices, chilies, corn and the beans into the saucepan and bring to boiling.

7. Adjust heat to low-heat and simmer without covering, for 60 minutes.

8. Serve chili into 8-10 bowls and top each bowl with a generous tablespoon of cheese.

9. Sprinkle fresh chopped cilantro over each chili bowl.

Roasted Turkey with Garlic Lime Dressing

Preparation Time: 15 minutes

Cook Time: 60 minutes

Serves: 4 servings

Ingredients

2 tbsps Dijon mustard

1/4 cup brown vinegar

2 chopped garlic cloves

2 tbsps fresh lime juice

Salt

2 tbsps olive oil

1 (4 lbs.) (chopped into smaller pieces) whole turkey

Freshly ground black pepper

1 tsp lime zest

1/2 cup chicken broth, low-salt

1 tbsp fresh parsley leaves, chopped

Instructions

1. Add pepper, salt, olive oil, garlic, lime juice, mustard and vinegar into a small bowl and mix until well combined.

2. Add turkey pieces and garlic lime dressing into a big ziplock bag.

3. Seal the bag and toss turkey mixture until well coated.

4. Place bag in a refrigerator for 2 hours or more.

TIP: Turn turkey pieces every now and then.

5. Heat up oven to 400°F.

6. Take out turkey from resealable bag and spread on a big pre-greased baking dish.

7. Transfer baking dish into the preheated oven and roast for about 60 minutes until just cooked through.

NOTE: Cover turkey with foil, if you discover it is browning speedily.

8. Place roasted turkey on a plate.

9. Add broth into the same baking dish over med-low heat.

10. Whisk pan drippings, chicken broth and any pan drippings until combined.

11. Drizzle sauce over turkey, sprinkled with parsley and lime zest.

Spicy and Healthy Saag Paneer

Preparation Time: 10 minutes

Cook Time: 18 minutes

Serves: 4 servings

Ingredients

¼ tsp ground turmeric

8 oz. (cut into 1/2" cubes) paneer cheese

1 (finely chopped) small onion

2 tbsps (divided) olive oil

1 minced garlic clove

1 (finely chopped) jalapeño pepper, if desired

2 tsps garam masala

1 tbsp fresh ginger, minced

20 oz. (thawed & finely chopped) frozen spinach

1 tsp cumin, ground

2 cups plain yogurt, low-fat

¾ tsp salt

Instructions

1. Add turmeric and paneer cheese into a fairly big bowl and toss until wholly coated.

2. Add 1 tbsp oil into a big nonstick skillet over med-heat.

3. Add paneer cheese into the hot oil and cook for about 5 minutes until browned on both sides, flip cheese once.

4. Place browned cheese in a plate.

5. Add the remaining 1 tbsp oil into the skillet.

6. Add jalapeno and onions into the skillet and stir cook for 7-8 minutes until golden brown.

TIP: Add a little water (2 tbsps at a time) into the skillet, if it looks dry while cooking.

7. Add cumin, garam masala, ginger and garlic into the skillet and stir cook for about 30 seconds until aromatic.

8. Add salt and spinach into the skillet mixture and stir for about 3 minutes until heated through.

9. Take skillet off heat, add paneer cheese and yogurt and stir until well incorporated.

10. Serve and enjoy.

Delicious Veggie Pad Thai

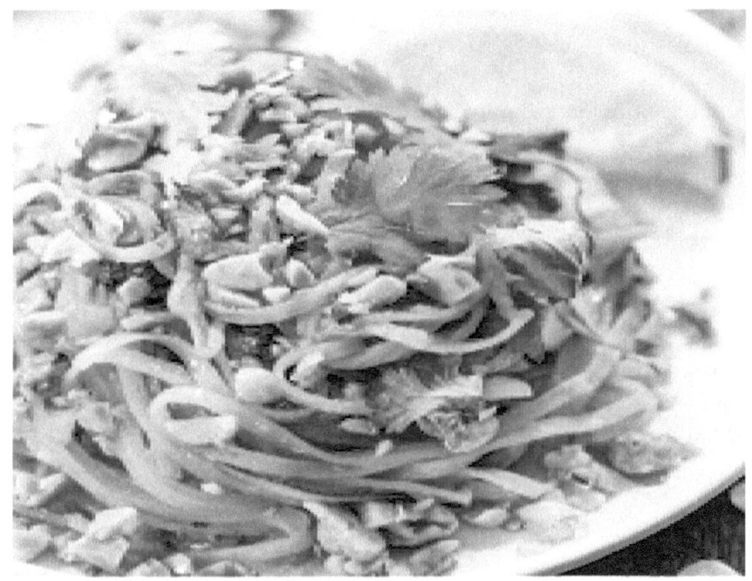

Preparation Time: 10 minutes

Cook Time: 30 minutes

Serves: 7-10 servings

Ingredients

1 (sliced into noodles with a veggie peeler or mandolin) large carrot

1 (sliced into noodles with a veggie peeler or mandolin) medium zucchini

½ cup purple cabbage, shredded

1 (chopped) green onion

½ cup mung bean sprouts

½ cup cauliflower florets

Sauce

2 tablespoons almond butter

2 tablespoons tahini

2 tablespoons wheat-free tamari

1 tablespoon lemon juice

¼ teaspoon minced garlic

1 tablespoon maple syrup

½ teaspoon grated ginger root

Instructions

1. Add zucchini and carrot noodles into a big bowl, topped with the other veggies.

2. Add sauce ingredients into a bowl and whisk until combined.

3. Pour almond butter sauce over veggies and noodles and toss until wholly coated.

4. Let sit until flavors are infused for 30 minutes.

5. Serve and eat.

Spiced Beef Tenderloin

Preparation Time: 5 minutes

Cook Time: 12 minutes

Serves: 4 servings

Ingredients

2 tablespoons garlic, minced

2 (discard stem, remove & chop leaves) fresh rosemary sprigs

2 teaspoons (dry toast lightly and grind) coriander seeds

1 teaspoon cinnamon

½ teaspoon allspice

2 teaspoons (dry toast lightly and grind) cumin seeds

½ teaspoon sea salt

1 teaspoon fresh ginger root, minced

4 (6 oz.) beef tenderloin filets

Instructions

1. Add salt, ginger root, spices, garlic and rosemary into a small bowl, combined and let sit until needed.

2. Transfer beef filets onto a 12"-by-12" baking dish and rub beef with the spice mix until evenly covered.

3. Heat up broiler on low-heat and generously moisten beef with broth or filtered water to prevent burning.

4. Broil beef tenderloins under the preheated broiler until beef is well cooked, for 4-6 minutes on each side.

TIP: Beef should be place 6" from the broiler

5. Take out beef from the oven and let sit until cooled before you serve.

Beverages

Lemony Avocado Protein Shake

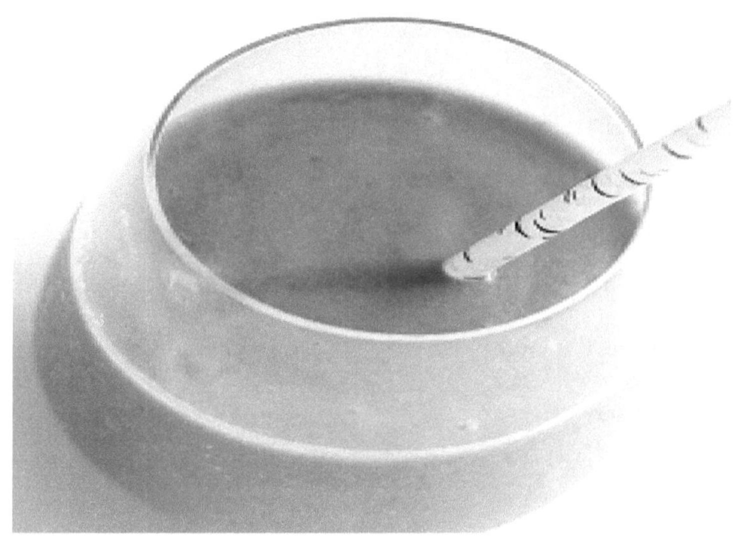

Preparation Time: 5 minutes

Cook Time: 0 minutes

Serves: 2 servings

Ingredients

2 scoops protein powder

1 1/2 cup almond milk

1/2 avocado

2 tablespoons flax seeds

1 lemon, juiced

3 dates, pitted

2 teaspoon ginger, chopped

Instructions

1. Add every ingredient into a high speed electric blender.

2. Blend until a smooth consistency is reached.

3. Serve and enjoy.

Pineapple Power Smoothie

Preparation Time: 10 minutes

Cook Time: 0 minutes

Serves: 1 serving

Ingredients

2 cups kale

1 cup brewed green tea, cooled to room temperature

1/3 cup (peeled & sliced into big chunks) cucumber

1 cup pineapple chunks, frozen

½ medium (peeled) banana

½ cup mango chunks, frozen

¼ teaspoon turmeric, ground

½" (peeled & cut from the stalk) fresh ginger

1 scoop protein powder

3 (coarsely chopped) mint leaves

4-5 ice cubes

1 tablespoon chia seeds

Instructions

1. Add every ingredient into a high speed electric blender, excluding the chia seeds.

2. Blend mixture until a smooth consistency is reached.

3. Add in the chia seeds into the blended mixture and process until incorporated and combined.

4. Serve and enjoy.

Hot Chocolate

Preparation Time: 5 minutes

Cook Time: 0 minutes

Serves: 1 serving

Ingredients

1/2 tsp cinnamon

1 tbsp raw cacao powder

1/2 tsp turmeric, dried

1/4 tsp ginger, dried

1 pinch cardamom, if desired

1 pinch cayenne pepper

1 pinch sea salt

1/2 tsp rice malt syrup

1/2 cup warmed coconut milk

1 pinch freshly ground black pepper

1/2 cup water

Instructions

1. Add pepper, sea salt, dried spices and raw cacao powder into a regular mug.

2. Add rice malt syrup and boiling water into the mug until filled halfway.

3. Stir mug mixture until combined and dissolved.

4. Add warm coconut milk into the mug and stir until evenly distributed.

5. Serve and enjoy.

Delicious Blueberry Smoothie

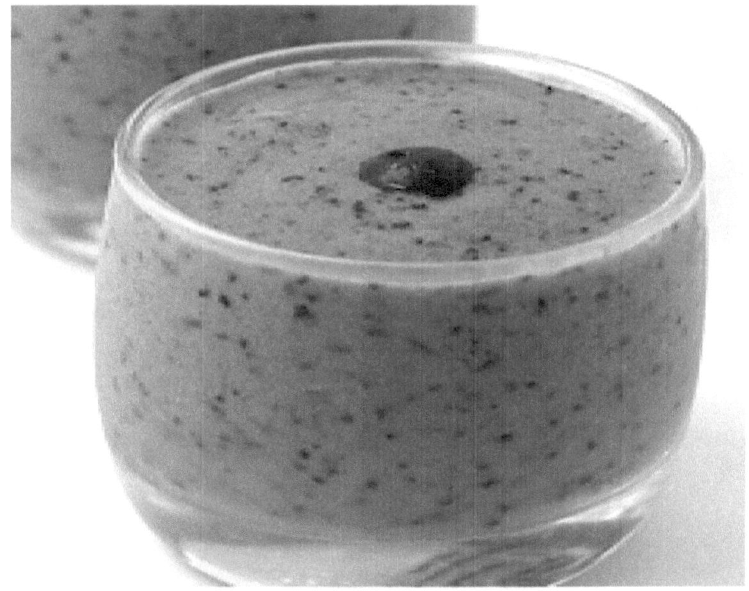

Preparation Time: 5 minutes

Cook Time: 0 minutes

Serves: 1 serving

Ingredients

1 banana, frozen

2 handfuls spinach

1 tablespoon almond butter

1/2 cup blueberries, frozen

1/8 - 1/4 teaspoon cayenne

1/4 teaspoon cinnamon

1/2 cup water

1 teaspoon maca powder, if desired

1/2 cup almond milk, unsweetened

Instructions

1. Add every ingredient into a high speed electric blender.

2. Process mixture until a smooth consistency is reached.

3. Serve and enjoy.

Ginger Root Tea

Preparation Time: 5 minutes

Cook Time: 10 minutes

Serves: 1 serving

Ingredients

1/4" slice ginger root

1 cup water

3 mint leaves

1 lime wedge, juiced

Instructions

1. Add water into a saucepan over med-high heat.

2. Bring water to boiling.

3. Add mint leaves, lime juice and ginger into a teacup.

4. Pour boiling water into the cup and stir to combine.

5. Serve and enjoy.

Avocado-Spinach Smoothie

Preparation Time: 5 minutes

Cook Time: 0 minutes

Serves: 1 serving

Ingredients

1 cup fresh spinach

1 cup plain yogurt, nonfat

¼ avocado

1 banana, chilled

1 tsp maple syrup

2 tbsps water

Instructions

1. Add maple syrup, water, avocado, banana, spinach and yogurt into a high speed electric blender.

2. Puree avocado and banana mixture until a smooth consistency is reached.

3. Serve and enjoy.

Healthy Turmeric Latte

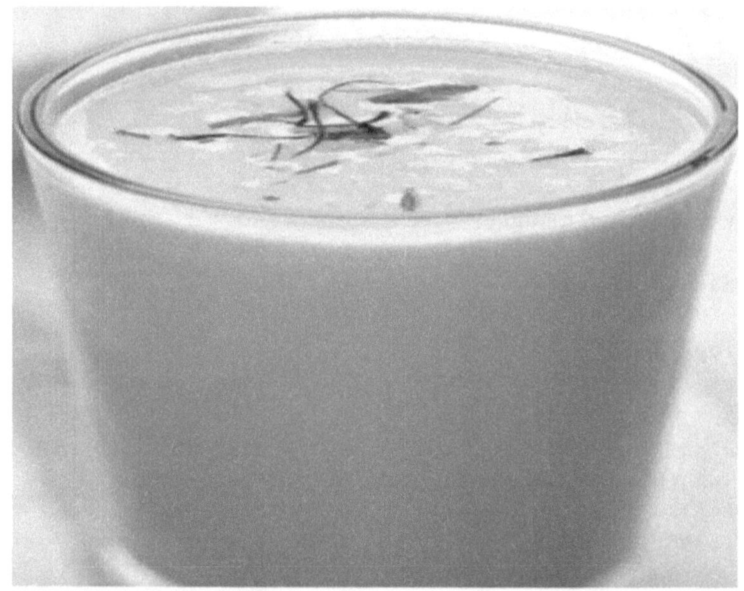

Preparation Time: 5 minutes

Cook Time: 5 minutes

Serves: 1 serving

Ingredients

1 tbsp fresh turmeric, grated

1 cup almond milk, unsweetened

1 tsp fresh ginger, grated

2 tsps honey

1 pinch of ground pepper

Garnish with

Cinnamon, ground

Instructions

1. Add pepper, ginger, honey, turmeric and milk into a high speed electric blender.

2. Blend mixture for about a minute, until a very smooth consistency is reached.

3. Pour the blended mixture into a saucepan over med-high heat.

4. Cook mixture until steaming hot and pour into a mug.

5. Garnish latter with cinnamon.

Chamomile Herbal Health Boost

Preparation Time: 20 minutes

Cook Time: 0 minutes

Serves: 4 servings

Ingredients

6 bags chamomile tea

4 cups boiling water

4 lime slices

2 tsps fresh ginger, grated

2 (lightly bruised) rosemary sprigs

2-4 tsps honey

Instructions

1. Add rosemary, honey, lime, ginger, chamomile tea bags and boiling water into a big oven secure bowl.

2. Stir until combined and let sit for 20 minutes until flavors are infused.

NOTE: Stir mixture every now and then.

3. Strain the rosemary mixture through a fine mesh sieve to get out as much liquid as you can.

TIP: Press on the tea bags until liquid is completely released.

4. Serve and enjoy.

Honeyed Matcha Green Tea Latte

Preparation Time: 2 minutes

Cook Time: 8 minutes

Serves: 1 serving

Ingredients

1 tsp matcha tea powder

¼ cup boiling water

1 tsp honey

1 cup milk, low-fat

Instructions

1. Add matcha powder and boiling water into a high speed electric blender.

2. Blend mixture until a foamy consistency is reached.

3. Add honey and milk into a pot and bring to just boiling.

4. Whisk the milk mixture energetically.

5. Transfer milk into a mug and add the blended tea.

6. Serve and enjoy.

Delicious Pineapple Smoothie

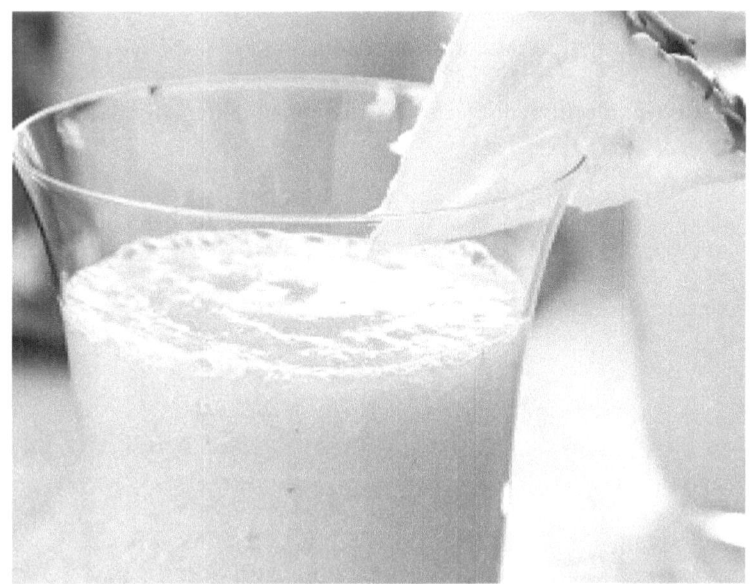

Preparation Time: 5 minutes

Cook Time: 0 minutes

Serves: 1 serving

Ingredients

1 (peeled) orange

1 ½ cups pineapple chunks, frozen

1 tbsp fresh ginger, finely-chopped

1 cup coconut water

1 tsp ground turmeric

1 tsp chia seeds

1/4 tsp black pepper, ground

Instructions

1. Add every ingredient into a high speed electric blender.

2. Process mixture until a smooth consistency is reached.

3. Serve and optionally garnish with any remaining chia seeds.

Grapefruit and Pineapple Green Smoothie

Preparation Time: 5 minutes

Cook Time: 0 minutes

Serves: 1 serving

Ingredients

1 small handful of (frozen, no-sugar) pineapple

1/2 a (frozen) grapefruit

1 small piece of fresh ginger root, peeled

1 large handful of fresh spinach

1 pinch cilantro

1 small piece of fresh turmeric root, peeled

1 scoop vanilla protein powder

1 celery stalk

Water

Instructions

1. Add every ingredient into a high speed electric blender.

2. Blend until a smooth consistency forms.

3. Serve and enjoy.

Desserts

Cheesecake Yogurt Cups

Preparation Time: 10 minutes

Cook Time: 2 minutes

Serves: 8 (1 cup) servings

Ingredients

2/3 cup cream cheese, reduced-fat

2 cups chocolate chips, semisweet

1/3 cup Greek yogurt, plain

1/4 cup powdered sugar

1/2 teaspoon fresh orange zest

Instructions

1. Add 1 1/2 cup chocolate chips into a oven-safe glass bowl.

2. Place glass bowl in a microwave and melt for 2 minutes, until wholly melted and smooth.

NOTE: Stir chocolate chips, once every 30 seconds

3. Add the reserved 1/2 cup chocolate chips into the glass bowl and stir until incorporated, glossy and smooth.

4. Add a dollop of melted chocolate into eight cupcake liners.

5. Spread chocolate evenly round each cupcake liner, filling the sides and evenly covering the bottom.

6. Place chocolate covered cupcake liners into a refrigerator.

7. In the meantime, add 1/4 cup powdered sugar and cream cheese into a fairly big bowl and beat until combined and smooth.

8. Add orange zest and Greek yogurt into the sugar and cream cheese mixture and mix until fully incorporated.

9. Add 1 spoonful of the sugar and cream cheese mixture into the set chocolate cups.

10. Spread cream cheese filling into one equal layer.

11. Return filled cups into the refrigerator until cheesecake firms up slightly, for about 5 minutes.

12. Stir the reserved melted chocolate and drizzle over cheesecake filling, carefully spreading chocolate over filling.

NOTE: If you have to, melt chocolate again for some seconds.

13. Return cups into the refrigerator until the chocolate has hardened, for 5-10 minutes.

14. Take out cheesecake from the liners, serve and enjoy.

Delicious Key Lime Pie

Preparation Time: 20 minutes

Cook Time: 0 minutes

Serves: 8 servings

Ingredients (Crust)

1 cup walnuts

1 cup shredded coconut, unsweetened

½ cup Medjool dates, pitted

¼ teaspoon sea salt

Fill with

3 tablespoons lime juice

3 firm avocados

½ cup raw honey

1 teaspoon lime zest

Lime slices

1 pinch sea salt

Instructions

1. Add salt, walnuts and coconut into a food processor.

2. Process mixture until a roughly ground consistency is reached.

3. Add dates into the processor and process until breadcrumb-like consistency is reached.

4. Pour mixture into a 9" pie plate and press with the back of a spatula.

5. Transfer crust into a freezer until chilled for 15 minutes.

6. Add every filling ingredient into a food processor and process until a smooth consistency is reached.

7. Pour blended filling mixture into the crust and return into the refrigerator for 20 minutes.

8. Serve garnished with thin fresh lime slices.

Pistachio Silky Chocolate Kiwi

Preparation Time: 5 minutes

Cook Time: 0 minutes

Serves: 1 serving

Ingredients

2 tsps dark chocolate, melted

1 (sliced) kiwi

1½ tsps salted roasted pistachios, chopped

Instructions

1. Drizzle melted chocolate over kiwi slices until wholly coated.

2. Top chocolate covered kiwi with a generous sprinkle of pistachios.

3. Serve and enjoy.

Salad

Pistachios, Cheese, Tangerine and Roasted Beet Salad

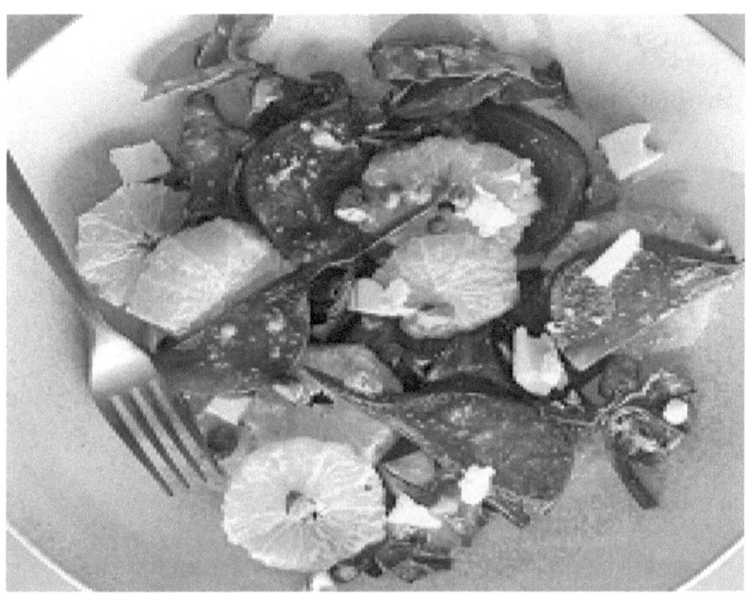

Preparation Time: 30 minutes

Cook Time: 1 hour 20 minutes

Serves: 4 servings

Ingredients

4 cups beet greens, chopped

2 (trimmed) medium beets

1 tbsp sherry vinegar

8 Pixie tangerines (1/2 tsp zest grated from 1 tangerine)

½ tsp (divided) kosher salt

¼ tsp Dijon mustard

6 tsps (divided) olive oil

Ground pepper, as needed

¼ cup toasted unsalted pistachios, roughly chopped

¼ cup feta cheese, crumbled

Instructions

1. Heat up oven to 375°F.

2. Wash beets thoroughly and wrap wet beet with aluminum foil.

3. Transfer foil wrapped beets into a small baking pan and transfer into the preheated oven.

4. Bake for 60-75 minutes, until a knife tip inserted into beet penetrates easily.

5. After baking, set wrapped beets aside for 15 minutes before unwrapping.

6. Let unwrapped beets sit for 10 more minutes until cooled.

7. Rub off beet skins using kitchen paper and trim beet ends off.

8. Cut beets into small slices.

9. Wash beet greens, drain, leave washed beet greens to be slightly damp and let sit until needed.

10. Slice off tangerine ends, and then remove white pith with the peel.

11. Slice tangerines into slices or segments and let sit until needed.

12. Add 1/4 tsp salt, mustard, vinegar, tangerine zest and generous pinch of ground pepper into a fairly big bowl.

13. Add 4 tsp oil into the zest mixture and whisk until combined.

14. Add sliced beets into the mixture, toss until coated and set aside until flavors are infused for 15 minutes.

15. Add the remaining 2 tsps oil into a big nonstick skillet over med-heat.

16. Add the greens into the hot oil and add 1/4 tsp salt.

17. Gently stir and cook for 2-3 minutes until just wilted.

18. Split greens into salad platters, topped with toasted pistachios, cheese, tangerine segments or slices and the beets.

19. Dribble any reserved dressing over salad and enjoy.

Delicious Grilled Eggplant Salad with Avocado

Preparation Time: 15 minutes

Cook Time: 10 minutes

Serves: 4 servings

Ingredients

1 (cut into rounds) big red onion

1 (cut into 1" thick slices) eggplant

1 (halved, pitted, peeled & chopped) avocado

Canola oil

1 tsp Dijon mustard

1 tbsp red wine vinegar

Maple syrup

1 tbsp oregano leaves, roughly chopped

Salt

Olive oil

1 lime, zested

Freshly ground black pepper

Parsley sprigs

Instructions

1. Coat red onions and eggplant with just enough canola oil.

2. Spread eggplant mixture on the grill.

3. Grill until onions are slightly charred and eggplants are tender.

4. Transfer eggplants and onions to a cutting board and let sit until slightly cooled.

5. Coarsely chop eggplants and onions and transfer into a serving bowl.

6. Add chopped avocado into the serving bowl and toss to combine.

7. Add oregano, Dijon and vinegar into a small bowl and whisk until combined.

8. Add olive oil and maple syrup into the small bowl and stir until dressing emulsifies.

9. Sprinkle dressing with pepper and salt.

10. Add dressing into the eggplant salt, garnished with parsley sprigs and lime zest.

Maple Walnuts, Cheese with Red Cabbage Salad

Preparation Time: 10 minutes

Cook Time: 7 minutes

Serves: 8 servings

Ingredients

¼ cup (divided) olive oil + 1 tbsp

1/3 cup + 1 tbsp blue cheese, crumbled

1 tbsp Dijon mustard

3 tbsps red-wine vinegar

¼ tsp pepper, freshly ground

¼ tsp salt

1 cup walnuts

1 tsp unsalted butter

¼ tsp freshly ground pepper

¼ tsp salt

8 cups red cabbage, sliced very thin

3 tbsps pure maple syrup

2 (sliced thin) scallion

Instructions

1. Add pepper, salt, mustard, vinegar, 1/4 cup oil, 1 tbsp blue cheese into small electric blender and process until a creamy texture forms.

2. Let pureed blue cheese dressing sit until needed.

3. Add butter and 1 tbsp oil into a fairly big skillet and heat.

NOTE: Place parchment paper piece near the stove.

4. Add walnuts into the hot oil and stir cook for 2 minutes.

5. Season with pepper and salt and dribble maple syrup over walnuts.

6. Stir cook for 3-5 minutes until nuts are well covered and just caramelized.

7. Place caramelized walnuts on parchment paper.

8. Scoop any remaining syrup over walnuts.

9. Break walnuts up while warm and let sit for 5 minutes until cooled.

10. Add scallions and cabbage into a big bowl and toss with the reserved blue cheese dressing.

11. Serve salad and top with the walnuts and remaining blue cheese.

Delicious Kale Salad

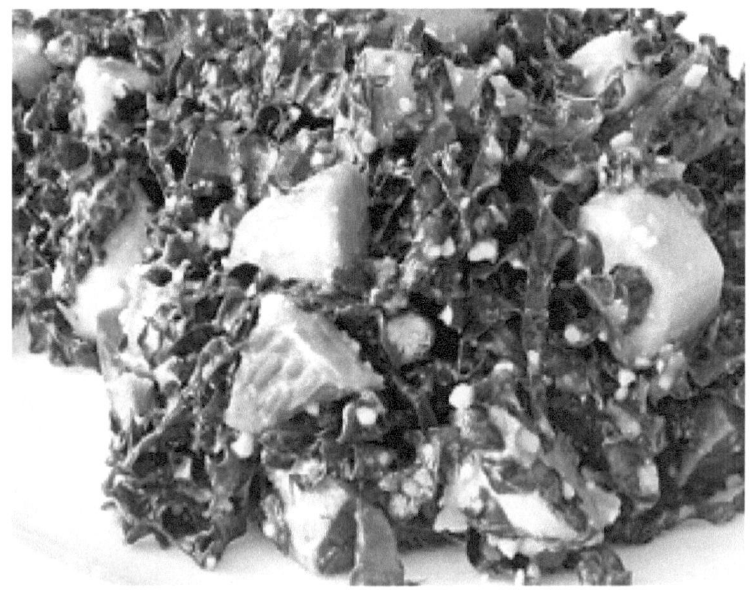

Preparation Time: 5 minutes

Cook Time: 7 minutes

Serves: 4 servings

Ingredients

½ lime

6 cups (washed & chopped) kale

1 pinch sea salt

1 pinch dried basil

2 tablespoons minced red onion

1 tablespoon olive oil

1 (sliced thin) small cucumber

2 tablespoons chopped green onion

¼ cup kalamata olives, chopped

1 minced garlic clove

Instructions

1. Add kale into a steamer basket and steam for 5-7 minutes.

2. Add kale, oil, salt, basil and lime into a big bowl and toss until evenly coated.

3. Add every other ingredient and mix until evenly distributed.

4. Serve at once and enjoy.

Blueberry Dressing with Green Salad

Preparation Time: 5 minutes

Cook Time: 0 minutes

Serves: 4 servings

Ingredients

1 tbsp brown rice vinegar

2 tsps blueberry jam

Salt and pepper, as needed

3 tbsps olive oil

4-5 cups romaine, chopped

1 pint (sliced) blueberries

Instructions

1. Add blueberry jam into a fairly big bowl.

2. Whisk in brown rice vinegar into the jam until incorporated.

3. Whisk in olive oil into the dressing mix and season with pepper and salt.

4. Add greens and blueberries into a bowl and toss until wholly coated with the dressing.

5. Serve and enjoy.

Ginger Dressed Spinach Salad

Preparation Time: 10 minutes

Cook Time: 0 minutes

Serves: 4 servings

Ingredients

3 tbsps olive oil

3 tbsps onion, minced

1½ tbsps fresh ginger, finely grated

2 tbsps white vinegar, distilled

1 tbsp soy sauce, reduced-sodium

1 tbsp ketchup

¼ tsp salt

¼ tsp garlic, minced

1 grated large carrot

Freshly ground pepper, as needed

10 oz. fresh spinach

1 (sliced very thin) medium red bell pepper

Instructions

1. Add pepper, salt, garlic, soy sauce, ketchup, ginger, vinegar, oil and onion into a high speed electric blender.

2. Blend mixture until a smooth consistency is reached.

3. Add bell pepper, carrot and spinach into a big bowl and toss with the blended dressing mixture until completely coated.

4. Serve and enjoy.

Olive Anchovy Salad with Orange

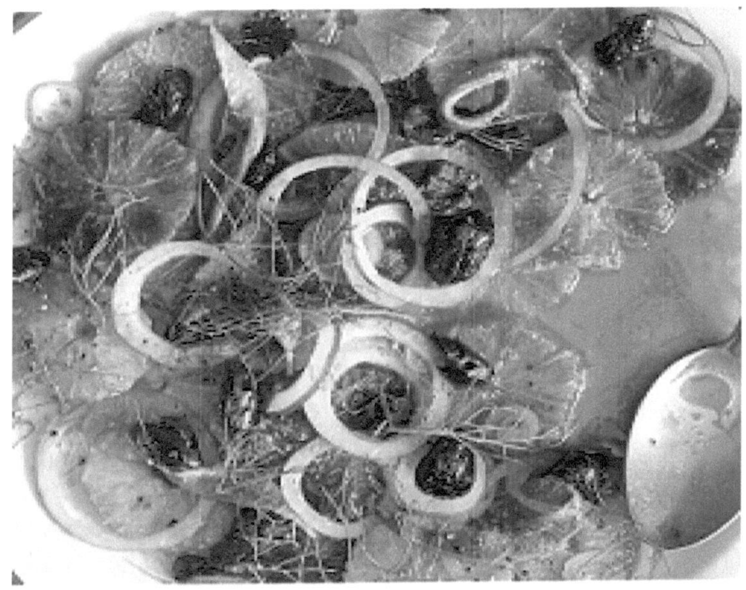

Preparation Time: 40 minutes

Cook Time: 0 minutes

Serves: 4 servings

Ingredients

1 (thinly sliced into circles) small red onion

4 small oranges

6 anchovy fillets

16 (pitted & halved) oil-cured Kalamata olives

3 tbsps olive oil

1 tbsp fresh lime juice

1/3 tsp ground pepper

Garnish with

2 tsps fennel fronds, finely minced

Instructions

1. Using a paring knife, peel the oranges.

2. Cut off the outside membrane covering the orange and white pith.

3. Cut orange into thin rounds.

NOTE: Make sure you save all the juice.

4. Place orange slices on a plate, keeping orange juice until needed.

5. Add anchovy fillets and olives on top of the orange rounds.

6. Drizzle oil and orange juice over salad and season with pepper.

7. Set salad aside until flavors are infused, for 30 minutes at room temperature.

8. Garnish salad and serve.

Beets Edamame with Green Salad

Preparation Time: 10 minutes

Cook Time: 0 minutes

Serves: 1 serving

Ingredients

1 cup (thawed) edamame, shelled

2 cups salad greens, mixed

1 tbsp red wine vinegar + 1½ tsps

½ medium (peeled & shredded) raw beet

2 tsps olive oil

1 tbsp fresh cilantro, chopped

Freshly ground pepper to taste

Salt

Instructions

1. Place beet, edamame and mixed salad greens on a big platter.

2. Add pepper, salt, oil, cilantro and vinegar into a small bowl and whisk dressing until combined.

3. Drizzle salad dressing over green salad mixture and toss until combined.

4. Serve and enjoy.

Blueberry, Peach and Watercress Salad with Bacon

Preparation Time: 10 minutes

Cook Time: 10 minutes

Serves: 4 servings

Ingredients (Bacon)

¼ cup port

8 oz. (slice crossways into 1/4" thick strips) bacon

1 tbsp pure maple syrup

¼ cup red wine

1½ tsps Chinese five-spice powder

2 peeled garlic cloves

Salad

2 tbsps olive oil

1 (sliced thin) medium shallot

1 tsp pure maple syrup

2 tbsps lemon juice

Pinch of sea salt

¼ tsp Chinese five-spice powder

3 (cut into 1/4" wedges) firm ripe peaches

¾ cup fresh blueberries

½ small head (separate the leaves and cut into 1" strips) radicchio

4 cups (tough stems trimmed) watercress

Instructions

1. Place a big skillet over med-heat.

2. Add bacon into the hot skillet and stir cook for 3-5 minutes until crisply browned.

3. Place browned bacon a plate lined with kitchen paper and get rid of bacon fat.

4. Place pan over high heat.

5. Add 1 1/2 tsps five spice powder, garlic cloves, 1 tbsp maple syrup, wine and port into the hot pan.

6. Bring mixture to boiling.

7. Return bacon into the skillet and stir cook with the sauce for about 2-3 minutes until bacon is glazed and coated and sauce is wholly reduced.

8. Take skillet off heat and let sit until needed.

9. Add salt, 5-spice powder, syrup, oil, lemon juice and shallot into a big bowl and stir until combined.

10. Add the blueberries into the salad mixture and crush with the back end of a spatula.

11. Add radicchio, watercress and peaches into the salad bowl and toss to coat.

12. Serve salad with the glazed bacon and enjoy.

Yummy Purple Fruit Salad

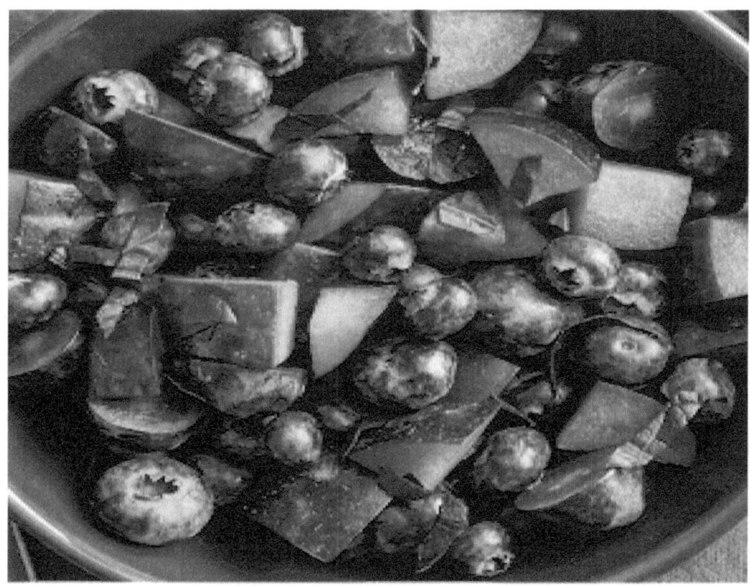

Preparation Time: 15 minutes

Cook Time: 0 minutes

Serves: 8 servings

Ingredients

2 cups blackberries

2 cups seedless black grapes, halved

2 tbsps purple basil, chopped (if desired)

2 cups plums, diced

Instructions

1. Add basil, plums, blackberries and grape into a big bowl.

2. Toss until combined.

3. Serve with desired dressing and enjoy.

Broccoli Slaw with Cabbage

Preparation Time: 15 minutes

Cook Time: 0 minutes

Serves: 6 servings

Ingredients

1 head cabbage, shredded

3 cups shredded broccoli

2 tbsps mayonnaise

1/4 cup nonfat Greek yogurt

1 tbsp fresh lime zest

1 tbsp lime juice, freshly squeezed

2 tsps maple syrup

1 tbsp lemon juice, freshly squeezed

1/8 cup fresh parsley leaves, chopped

1/2 tsp garlic seasoning

1 chopped green onion

Garlic Seasoning

1/4 cup pepper

1 cup salt

1/4 cup garlic powder

Instructions

1. Add garlic seasoning ingredients into a small bowl and mix well until combined.

2. Add the shredded cabbage and broccoli into a big bowl.

3. Add 1/2 tsp garlic seasoning, maple syrup, lemon, lime zest, lime juice, mayonnaise and yogurt into a bowl and whisk until combined.

4. Add dressing over broccoli slaw and toss until well coated.

5. Add green onions and parsley into the salad and toss until combined.

6. Place a lid over bowl and refrigerate for 60 minutes before you serve.

Spinach Tuna Salad

Preparation Time: 10 minutes

Cook Time: 0 minutes

Serves: 1 serving

Ingredients

1½ tbsps lime juice

1½ tbsps tahini

1 (5-oz.) can (drained) tuna in water

1½ tbsps water

2 tbsps feta cheese

4 (pitted and chopped) kalamata olives

2 cups baby spinach

2 tbsps parsley

1 (sliced) medium orange

Instructions

1. Add water, lime juice and tahini into a bowl and whisk until combined.

2. Stir in parsley, feta, olives and tuna into the bowl until combined.

3. Serve the tuna olives mixture over 2 cups of spinach.

4. Add sliced orange to the side and dig in.

Caramelized Onions, Sardines with Romaine Wedges

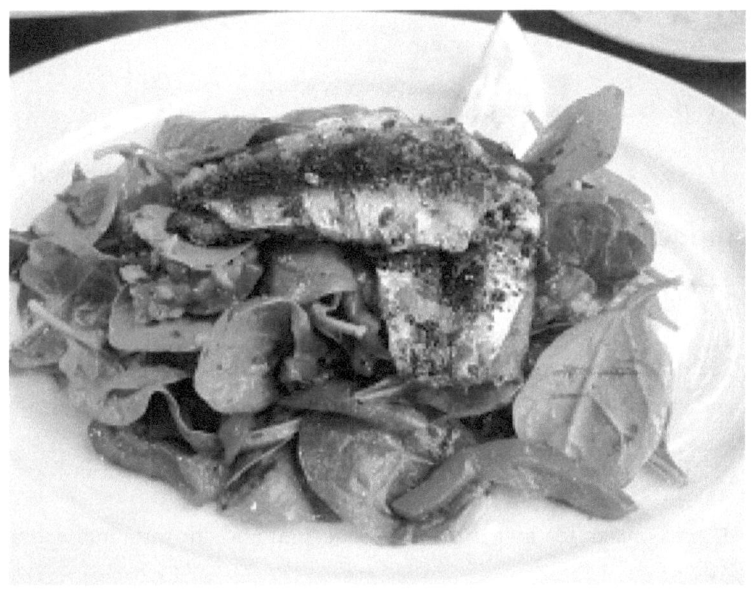

Preparation Time: 10 minutes

Cook Time: 20 minutes

Serves: 4 servings

Ingredients

1 (sliced) big sweet onion

1 tbsp extra-virgin olive oil

2 tbsps balsamic vinegar

1/3 tsp (divided) salt + ½ tsp

2 tbsps mayonnaise, low-fat

½ cup plain Greek yogurt, reduced-fat

4 tsps shallot, minced

2 tbsps white-wine vinegar

2 hearts (halved lengthways & cored) romaine

¼ tsp freshly ground pepper

1 cup cherry tomatoes

2 (4-oz.) cans {drained} sardines with bones, packed in olive oil

Instructions

1. Add oil into a small saucepan over med-heat.

2. Add 1/3 tsp salt and onion into the saucepan, place lid over saucepan and stir cook for 12-15 minutes, until onions are just brown and tender.

3. Adjust heat to med-low heat.

4. Add balsamic vinegar into the saucepan and stir until incorporated.

5. Remove lid from saucepan and simmer for 1-3 minutes until it is reduced to a glazed.

6. Add the remaining 1/2 tsp salt, pepper, shallot, white wine vinegar, mayonnaise and yogurt into a small bowl and whisk until combined.

7. Split romaine halves between four platters.

8. Scoop dressing/vinaigrette over each plate.

9. Split each sardine into 2-3 pieces and split between romaine halves.

10. Top each salad with tomatoes and the caramelized onions.

11. Serve and enjoy.

Delicious Chickpea Salad

Preparation Time: 10 minutes

Cook Time: 0 minutes

Serves: 4 servings

Ingredients

1 (grated) carrot

2 (19-oz.) can {drained & rinsed} chickpeas

1/2 (diced) green bell pepper

1/2 (diced) red onion

2 tbsps olive oil

1/4 cup lime juice

Freshly ground black pepper

Salt

1/4 cup parsley leaves, freshly chopped

Instructions

1. Add every ingredient into a big mixing bowl.

2. Toss chickpea mixture until combined.

3. Serve and enjoy.

Broccoli with Oven Roasted Garlic Salmon

Preparation Time: 10 minutes

Cook Time: 15 minutes

Serves: 4 servings

Ingredients

2 (washed & cut into florets) heads of broccoli

1 1/2 lbs. (skinned & sliced into 4 portions) salmon fillets

1-2 (divided) minced garlic cloves

3 tbsps melted coconut oil

1/2 tsp (divided) ground black pepper

1 1/4 tsp (divided) sea salt

1 sliced lime, if desired

Instructions

1. Heat up oven to 450°F.

2. Prepare a big parchment paper lined baking sheet.

3. Lay salmon portions on the prepared baking and leave room between each piece.

4. Dribble 1 tbsp oil over salmon portions.

5. Evenly spread minced garlic over fishes.

6. Season salmon with 1/4 tsp ground black pepper and 1/2 tsp salt.

7. Top fish with lime slices.

8. Add broccoli florets into a bowl and combined with 1/4 tsp ground black pepper, 3/4 tsp sea salt and 2 tbsps oil.

9. Toss until broccoli florets are evenly coated.

10. Lay seasoned florets around the fish portions on the baking sheet.

11. Transfer baking sheet into the preheated oven and bake until florets edges are just golden and the fish is well cooked, for 13-15 minutes.

12. Serve and enjoy.

Delicious Maple Brussels Sprouts Salmon

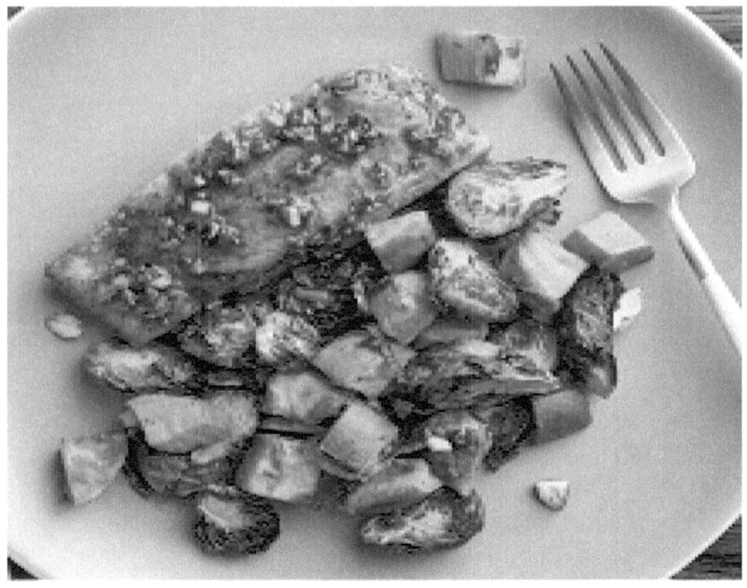

Preparation Time: 5 minutes

Cook Time: 25 minutes

Serves: 4 servings

Ingredients

16 ounces (halved) Brussels sprouts

4 (4-6 ounces) salmon filets with their skin on

1 (16 ounces) baby potatoes bag

1 bunch (trimmed & cut in 1/2) asparagus

1 cup cherry tomatoes

½ (cubed) red onion

2 tbsps maple syrup

2 tbsps olive oil

1 tbsp dijon mustard

3 tbsps brown rice vinegar

1 tsp fresh thyme

1 minced garlic clove

½ tsp sea salt

Instructions

1. Heat up oven to 450°F.

2. Add salt, thyme, garlic, dijon mustard, vinegar and maple syrup into a small bowl and whisk until combined.

3. Add olive oil, cherry tomatoes, red onion, baby potatoes, asparagus, and Brussels sprouts into a big bowl.

4. Add 3 tbsps maple syrup vinegar into the sprouts mixture and toss until well coated, using clean hands.

5. Spread veggies on a baking sheet in one layer and transfer into the preheated oven.

6. Bake veggies for 10 minutes and take baking pan out of the oven.

7. Lay fish fillets with the skin side down over the veggies.

NOTE: Leave 1" room between fish pieces.

8. Coat fillets with the maple vinegar mixture and return pan into the oven.

9. Bake for 10 more minutes.

10. Set broiler to high and brown fish top for 3-4 more minutes.

11. Take baking pan out of the oven, serve and enjoy.

Turmeric, Shrimp and Bok Choy Soup

Preparation Time: 20 minutes

Cook Time: 30 minutes

Serves: 4 servings

Ingredients

1 big chopped onion

1 tbsp olive oil

1 1/2 tsp salt

6 minced garlic cloves

1 tsp turmeric

1 tsp freshly ground black pepper

2 (sliced) carrots

6 cups chicken broth

6 heads (bottoms chopped off) baby bok choy

1 lb. (stems removed & sliced into 1/2" pieces) shitake mushrooms

1 lb. shrimp

Instructions

1. Add oil into a stock pot over med-heat.

2. Add garlic and onions into the hot oil and saute until translucent, for 5 minutes.

3. Add mushrooms, carrots, broth, turmeric, pepper and salt into the pot and bring to boiling.

4. Adjust heat to low heat, place lid over pot and simmer for 15 minutes.

5. Add shrimp and bok choy into the pot and simmer for 5 more minutes.

6. Season with pepper and salt, serve and enjoy.

Tuna Salad with Olives, Tomatoes and Mayo

Preparation Time: 15 minutes

Cook Time: 0 minutes

Serves: 2 servings

Ingredients

1/4 cup mayonnaise

2 (5 ounces) cans {drained} tuna packed in water

2 tbsps red onion, minced

1/4 cup kalamata olives, chopped

2 tbsps fresh basil, chopped

2 tbsps fire roasted red peppers, chopped

1 tbsp fresh lime juice

1 tbsp capers

2 (slice into sixths, do not cut all the way through) large tomatoes, vine-ripened

Salt and pepper

Instructions

1. Add every ingredient into a big bowl, excluding the tomatoes.

2. Stir mixture until combined.

3. Ladle tuna salad mixture into each opened tomato until filled.

4. Serve and enjoy.

Grilled Turkey Wrap with Kale Caesar Salad

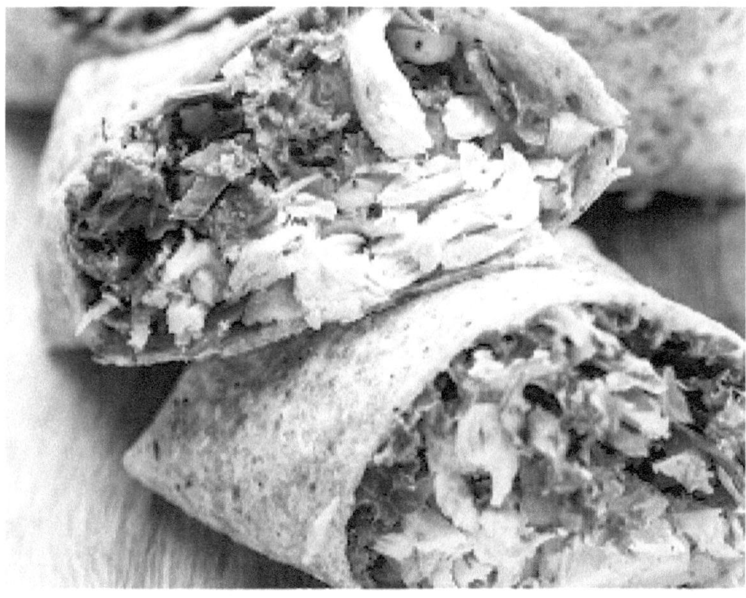

Preparation Time: 10 minutes

Cook Time: 0 minutes

Serves: 2 servings

Ingredients

6 cups (cut into bite sized pieces) curly kale

8 oz. (sliced thin) grilled turkey

3/4 cup Parmesan cheese, finely shredded

1 cup (quartered) cherry tomatoes

1 minced garlic clove

½ (cooked for 1 minute) coddled egg

1 tsp honey

1/2 tsp Dijon mustard

1/8 cup extra-virgin olive oil

1/8 cup fresh lime juice

2 big tortillas

Kosher salt and freshly ground black pepper

Instructions

1. Add olive oil, lime juice, honey, mustard, minced garlic and 1/2 of the coddled egg into a bowl.

2. Whisk olive oil mixture until a dressing consistency is reached.

3. Sprinkle pepper and salt over dressing.

4. Add cherry tomatoes, grilled turkey and kale into a bowl and toss until combined.

5. Toss kale salad with 1/4 cup shredded parmesan and the dressing.

6. Generously scoop kale salad over tortillas and top each tortilla with 1/4 cup parmesan.

7. Roll up tortillas and slice in two.

8. Serve at once and enjoy.

Seafood

Lemon Ginger Sauce with Green Tea Poached Salmon

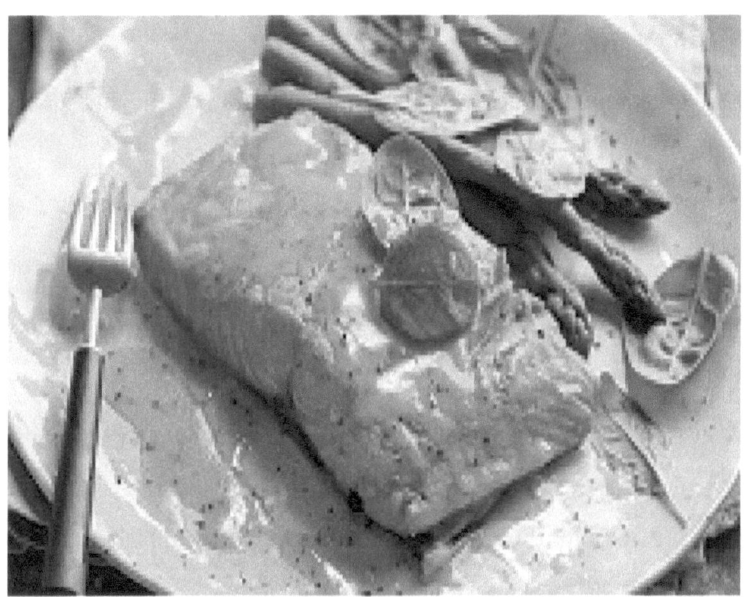

Preparation Time: 10 minutes

Cook Time: 30 minutes

Serves: 4 servings

Ingredients

2 (halved) lemons

10 cups water

4" piece (peeled & chopped) fresh ginger

6 tbsps (divided) maple syrup

2 tsps whole black peppercorns

2 tsps sea salt

4 (6 oz.) salmon fillets, boneless skinless

4-6 tbsps loose green tea

Instructions

1. Add water into a well lidded pot.

2. Add 3 lemon halves into the pot with their juices freshly squeezed into the water.

3. Add peppercorns, salt, ginger and 5 tbsps maple syrup into the pot.

4. Bring mixture to boiling over med-high heat.

5. Lower heat, place lid over pot and simmer until flavors are infused, for 10 minutes.

6. Take out 1/2 cup of poaching juice from the pot and reserve for later use.

7. Take pot with the remaining poaching juice from heat and stir in the tea.

8. Let poaching juice and tea mixture sit until flavors are infused, for 3-5 minutes.

9. Gently add fillets into the hot tea with poaching juice mixture.

10. Place lid over pot and poach salmon for about 6-7 minutes, until fillets are firm and cooked through.

11. In the meantime, add 1 tbsp maple syrup, the zest of remaining lemon half, the reserved poaching juice into a small pot over low heat.

12. Simmer poaching juice mixture for about 7-10 minutes, until juice is thickened and reduced by 2/3.

13. Using a slotted spoon, remove poached salmon and place on serving plates, drizzled with bit of simmered sauce.

Brussels Sprouts and Roasted Salmon with Garlic

Preparation Time: 10 minutes

Cook Time: 25 minutes

Serves: 6 servings

Ingredients

¼ cup olive oil

14 big (divided) garlic cloves garlic

1 tsp (divided) salt

2 tbsps (divided) fresh oregano, finely chopped

6 cups (trimmed & sliced) Brussels sprouts

¾ tsp (divided) freshly ground pepper

2 lbs. (skinned & cut into 6 portions) wild-caught salmon fillet

¾ cup white wine

Lime wedges

Instructions

1. Heat up oven to 450°F.

2. Add 1/4 tsp pepper, 1/2 tsp salt, 1 tbsp oregano, oil and 2 minced garlic cloves into a bowl and combine.

3. Halve the remaining garlic cloves.

4. Add 3 tbsps of the oil and seasoning mixture, the Brussels sprouts and garlic halves into a big roasting pan and toss until combined.

5. Place pan into the preheated oven and roast for 15 minutes and stir once.

6. Add white wine into the remaining seasoning oil mixture and combine.

7. Take out roasting pan from the oven, stir the veggies and top with the fish portions.

8. Dribble the oil seasoning and wine mixture over the veggies and salmon mixture in the pan.

9. Sprinkle pan mixture with 1/2 tsp pepper, 1/2 tsp salt and the remaining 1 tbsp oregano.

10. Return roasting pan into the oven and roast for 5-10 more minutes until fish is cooked through.

11. Serve, topped with lime wedges.

Bagna Cauda Veggies with Salmon

Preparation Time: 15 minutes

Cook Time: 25 minutes

Serves: 4 servings

Ingredients

1 bunch (trimmed) broccolini

1 lb. (cut into 1/2" thick wedges) sweet potato

½ tsp (divided) salt

1 tbsp olive oil

1 small (cut into 1/2" thick wedges and reserve fronds) fennel bulb

1 lb. salmon

½ small head (cut into 1/2" thick wedges) radicchio

2 fairly big heads (separate the leaves) Belgian endive

Bagna Cauda

2 (sliced very thin) garlic cloves

1/3 cup olive oil

2 tbsps sherry vinegar

8 anchovy fillets

1 tbsp butter

Instructions

1. Heat up oven to 425°F.

2. Prepare a big rimmed cooking spray covered baking sheet.

3. Add broccolini and sweet potato wedges into a big bowl.

4. Sprinkle broccolini mixture with 1/4 tsp salt and 1 tbsp oil and toss until combined.

5. Spread sweet potato wedges onto the coated baking sheet.

TIP: Leave the broccolini until later.

6. Transfer baking sheet into the preheated oven and roast for 15 minutes, flipping once while roasting.

7. Push roasted sweet potatoes to a side of the baking sheet until a hole is made at the center.

8. Place salmon at center of the baking pan seasoned with the remaining 1/4 tsp salt.

9. Spread broccolini just about the salmon and return baking sheet into the oven.

10. Roast salmon mixture for 6-10 minutes, until salmon is just cooked through and the veggies are softened.

11. In the meantime, add oil into a small saucepan over med-low heat.

12. Add garlic into the oil and cook for about 2 minutes until aromatic.

13. Add the anchovies into the saucepan and light crush with the back end of a spatula until they flake apart.

14. Add butter and vinegar into the saucepan, stir cook over very low heat for 2 more minutes.

15. Place broccolini, sweet potatoes and salmon on a serving platter.

16. Layer salmon mixture with radicchio, endive and fennel.

17. Garnish dish with the reserved fronds.

18. Drizzle with bagna cauda and dig in.

Dill Dressed Salmon with Cucumbers and Tomatoes

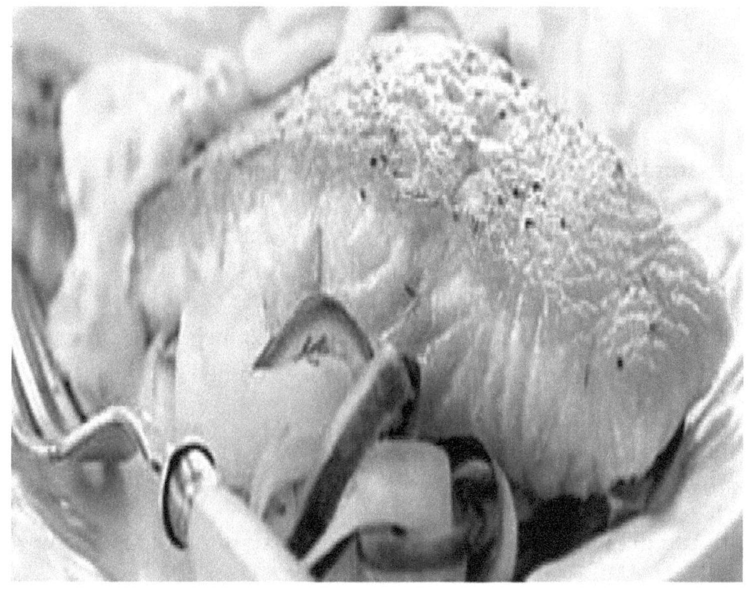

Preparation Time: 10 minutes

Cook Time: 15 minutes

Serves: 4 servings

Ingredients

2 (seeded & diced) small plum tomatoes

1/2 (diced into 1/4" pieces) cucumber, seedless

2 tbsps Dijon mustard

1 (finely chopped) shallot

1/4 cup white wine vinegar

2 tbsps maple syrup

1/4 cup fresh dill, finely chopped

1/2 cup olive oil

Freshly ground black pepper

Salt

4 (6 oz.) salmon fillets, skinless

Instructions

1. Add 1/2 of the shallots, diced tomatoes and cucumbers into a bowl and combine.

2. Add the reserved shallot half, white wine vinegar, maple syrup and mustard into a small bowl and whisk until combined.

3. Add in olive oil into the mustard dressing in a slow and steady stream while whisking.

4. Add dill into the dressing mixture and stir until incorporated.

5. Sprinkle pepper and salt over dressing.

6. Sprinkle black pepper and salt over salmon.

7. Add olive oil into a nonstick skillet over med-high heat.

8. Add the seasoned fish into the hot oil with the rounded side down.

9. Cook fish for 3-4 minutes until edges are slightly crispy and the fish is golden.

10. Flip fish over and cook until fish is opaque for 4 minutes.

11. Split salmon into serving platter, topped with tomato, cucumbers and shallot mixture and generous scoops of dill dressing.

12. Serve and enjoy.

Cauliflower Rice with Salmon Bowl

Preparation Time: 10 minutes

Cook Time: 35 minutes

Serves: 2 servings

Ingredients

10-12 (chopped in /2) Brussels sprouts

2 organic salmon fillets

½ (riced in a food processor) head cauliflower

1 (cleaned & shredded) bunch kale

1 tsp curry powder

3 tbsps (divided) olive oil

Salt

Marinade

1 tsp Dijon mustard

¼ cup tamari sauce

1 tsp maples syrup, if desired

1 tsp sesame oil

1 tbsp sesame seeds

Instructions

1. Heat up oven to 350°F.

2. Prepare a parchment paper lined baking tray.

3. Add Brussels sprouts onto the prepared baking tray and cover 1 tbsp olive oil.

4. Sprinkle salt over oil coated sprouts and place in the preheated oven for 20 minutes until roasted.

5. In the meantime, add every marinade ingredient into a bowl and whisk until combined.

6. After roasting, add salmon fillets into the baking tray.

7. Generously scoop marinade over fillets and return sprouts and the fillets into the oven.

8. Roast until salmon is well cooked, for 13-15 more minutes.

9. In the meantime, add 1 tbsp olive oil into a skillet over med-high heat.

10. Add kale into the hot oil and saute for 2-3 minutes until wilted.

11. Take out kale and let sit until needed.

12. Add the remaining tablespoon olive oil into the skillet.

13. Add cauliflower rice into the hot oil, seasoned with salt and 1 tsp curry powder.

14. Saute cauliflower rice for 2-3 minutes until cooked.

15. Take out Brussels sprouts and the fillets from the oven and split evenly into 2 serving bowls.

16. Add sautéed cauliflower rice and kale to the salmon mixture.

17. Toss to combine, serve and enjoy.

Rosemary Pecan Topping with Baked Tilapia

Preparation Time: 15 minutes

Cook Time: 18 minutes

Serves: 4 servings

Ingredients

1/3 cup panko breadcrumbs, whole wheat

1/3 cup raw pecans, chopped

1/2 teaspoon brown sugar

2 teaspoon fresh rosemary, chopped

1 pinch cayenne pepper

1/8 teaspoon salt

1 egg white

1 1/2 teaspoon extra-virgin olive oil

4 (4 ounce each) tilapia fillets

Instructions

1. Heat up oven to 350°F.

2. Add cayenne pepper, salt, brown sugar, rosemary, breadcrumbs and pecans into a small baking dish and stir until combined.

3. Add olive into the pecan mixture and toss until wholly coated.

4. Transfer baking dish into the preheated oven and bake for 7-8 minutes until light golden brown.

5. Adjust oven temperature to 400°F.

6. Coat a big glass baking sheet with cooking spray until well covered.

7. Add egg white into a shallow dish and whisk.

8. Dip fillets in the egg mixture and then immerse in the pecan mixture until every side is lightly coated.

NOTE: Work in batches.

9. Transfer the coated fish fillets into the sprayed glass baking dish.

10. Add the remaining pecan mixture over fillets and press.

11. Place baking sheet into the preheated oven and bake for about 10 minutes, until fillets is just cooked through.

12. Serve and enjoy.

Greens, Chickpeas with Roasted Salmon

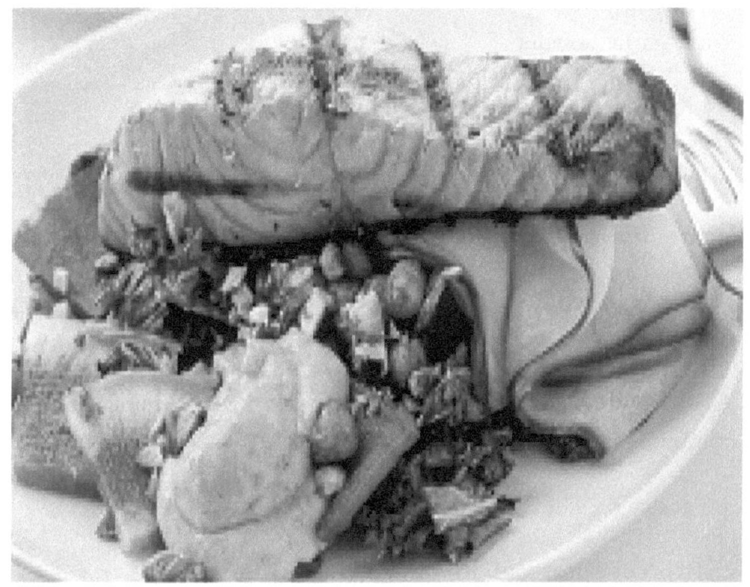

Preparation Time: 10 minutes

Cook Time: 40 minutes

Serves: 4 servings

Ingredients

1 tbsp paprika, smoked

2 tbsps (divided) olive oil

1 (15 oz.) can (rinsed) chickpeas, no-salt-added

½ tsp (divided) salt

¼ cup mayonnaise

1/3 cup buttermilk

½ tsp (divided) ground pepper

¼ cup fresh chives, chopped + more for garnish

10 cups kale, chopped

¼ tsp garlic powder

1¼ lbs. (cut into 4 portions) wild salmon

¼ cup water

Instructions

1. Heat up oven to 425°F with racks positioned in middle and upper third of the oven.

2. Add 1/4 tsp salt, paprika and 1 tbsp oil into a fairly big bowl and combine.

3. Pat dry the chickpeas until meticulously dried.

4. Toss chickpeas with the salt and oil mixture.

5. Pour seasoned chickpeas on a rimmed baking sheet and spread.

6. Transfer baking sheet into the upper rack of the preheated oven.

7. Roast chickpeas for 30 minutes, stirring two times.

8. In the meantime, add garlic powder, 1/4 tsp pepper, herbs, mayonnaise and buttermilk into a high speed electric blender and puree until a smooth consistency is reached.

9. Let pureed buttermilk mixture sit until needed.

10. Add the remaining 1 tbsp oil into a big skillet over med-heat.

11. Add kale into the hot oil and cook for 2 minutes, stirring every now and then.

12. Add water into the skillet and cook for about 5 more minutes until the kale is softened.

13. Take skillet off heat, add a pinch of salt, and stir until incorporated.

15. Take out baking sheet from the oven and push chickpeas to a side of the baking sheet.

16. Add salmon to the empty side of the baking sheet, seasoned with 1/4 tsp pepper and 1/4 tsp salt.

17. Return baking sheet into the oven and bake for about 5-8 minutes, until the fish is just cooked through.

18. Drizzle the buttermilk dressing over salmon, garnished with additional herbs, if desired.

19. Serve salmon with roasted chickpeas and kale.

20. Enjoy.

Delicious Asian Grilled Mackerel

Preparation Time: 30 minutes

Cook Time: 7 minutes

Serves: 4 servings

Ingredients

1 tbsp olive oil

2 tbsps chile paste

2 tsps rice vinegar

1 tbsp soy sauce, reduced-sodium

2 (about 1.5 lbs each) whole mackerel

1 tsp fresh ginger, grated

Instructions

1. Clean and butterfly fish with leave their tails on

2. Add ginger, vinegar, soy sauce, oil and chile paste into a small bowl and whisk until a smooth consistency is reached.

3. Place 2 tbsps of the chile paste marinade into a separate small bowl and let sit for later use.

4. Expose the flesh of each butterflied fish and transfer onto a big baking sheet with the skin side down.

5. Spread the marinade over fish flesh until evenly covered.

6. Transfer fish into a refrigerator until marinated, for 30-60 minutes.

7. Heat up grill to high heat, about 20 minutes before grilling.

8. Add oil to a folded kitchen paper held with tongues and rub oiled kitchen paper over grill rack.

9. Place marinated fish over grill with the flesh side down and grill for 3 minutes.

10. Using a big spatula, flip fish over, spread the marinade kept back over the fish and grill for 3-4 more minutes, until opaque in the middle.

11. Serve and enjoy.

One Pan Zucchini and Lime Herb Salmon

Preparation Time: 15 minutes

Cook Time: 20 minutes

Serves: 4 servings

Ingredients

2 tbsps olive oil

4 chopped zucchini

Kosher salt and freshly ground black pepper, as necessary

Salmon

2 tbsps lime juice, freshly squeezed

2 tbsps packed brown sugar

2 minced garlic cloves

1 tbsp Dijon mustard

1/2 tsp oregano, dried

1/2 tsp dried dill

1/4 tsp rosemary, dried

1/4 tsp thyme, dried

4 (5-oz.) salmon fillets

Kosher salt and freshly ground black pepper, as needed

2 tbsps fresh parsley leaves, chopped

Instructions

1. Heat up oven to 400°F.

2. Lightly coat baking sheet with nonstick cooking spray.

3. Add rosemary, thyme, oregano, dill, garlic, Dijon, lime juice and brown sugar into a small bowl and whisk until combined.

4. Sprinkle pepper and salt over brown sugar mixture and let sit until needed.

5. Lay zucchini onto the sprayed baking sheet in one layer.

6. Dribble olive oil over zucchini and sprinkle with pepper and salt, as necessary.

7. Add salmon onto the baking sheet in one layer.

8. Brush each fish fillet with the lime herb mixture until wholly covered.

9. Transfer baking dish into the preheated oven and bake for about 16-18 minutes, until fillet flakes easily with a fork.

10. Serve and enjoy.

Potato and Smoked Salmon Tartine

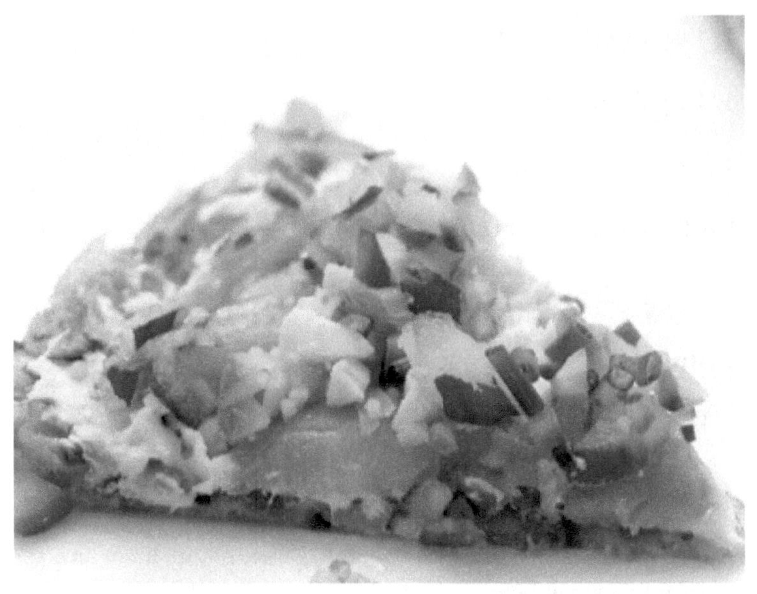

Preparation Time: 25 minutes

Cook Time: 20 minutes

Serves: 2 servings

Ingredients (Potato Tartine)

2 tbsps clarified butter

1 (peeled & grated lengthways) large russet potato

Kosher salt and freshly ground black pepper

Top with

1 1/2 tbsps chives, finely minced

4 oz. (at room temp) soft goat cheese

1/2 a lime, zested

1/2 (minced finely) garlic clove

2 tbsps capers, drained

Smoked salmon, sliced thin

1/2 (finely chopped) hardboiled egg

2 tbsps red onion, finely chopped

Garnish with

Chives, finely minced

Instructions

1. Add garlic, lime zest and goat cheese into a small bowl and combine.

2. Season cheese mixture with pepper and salt as desired.

3. Add fresh chives into the mixture and gently stir until incorporated.

4. Let cheese mixture sit until needed.

5. Sprinkle salt over hardboiled egg and chopped red onion.

6. Get rid of excess liquid by squeezing grated potatoes over the sink.

7. Liberally sprinkle pepper and salt over potatoes and toss until wholly coated.

8. Add clarified butter into a big skillet over med-high heat.

9. Add the grated potato into the hot oil.

10. Use a spatula to shape coarsely into one big circle.

11. Press potato circle with the back of a spatula until compact.

12. Place lid over skillet and cook until potato bottom is golden brown, for 8-10 minutes.

13. Carefully turn potato cake over and cook until crispy and golden brown, for 8-10 more minutes.

14. Let sit on a cooling rack until cooled.

15. Spread goat cheese mixture over potato cake.

16. Top with smoked salmon and sprinkle with the capers, hard-boiled egg and red onion.

17. Garnish with freshly chopped chives.

18. Cut cake into wedges and serve at once.

Side Dishes

Limey Ginger Turmeric Dressing

Preparation Time: 5 minutes

Cook Time: 0 minutes

Serves: 1/2 cup

Ingredients

1" (skin removed) fresh ginger

1/4 cup lime juice

2 tsp turmeric, ground

1 garlic clove

1 tbsp lemon juice

3 tbsps olive oil

Salt, as needed

1/4 tsp black pepper

Instructions

1. Add every ingredient into a high speed electric blender.

2. Blend until a smooth consistency is reached.

3. Check for and adjust seasoning as necessary.

4. Serve over roasted veggies, protein and salads.

Chickpeas with Roasted Cauliflower

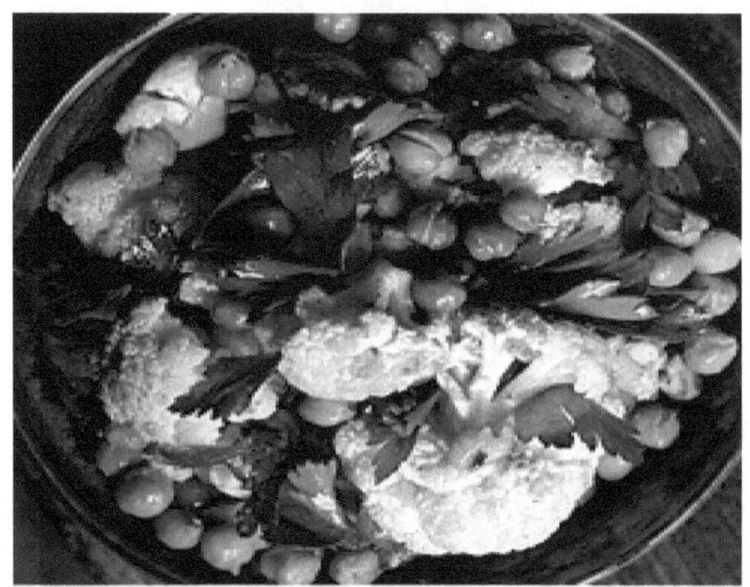

Preparation Time: 10 minutes

Cook Time: 25 minutes

Serves: 3-4 servings

Ingredients

1 1/2 cups chickpeas, cooked

1 head (cut into florets) cauliflower

2 minced garlic cloves

3 tbsp olive oil

1 tsp cumin, ground

1 1/2 tsps turmeric, ground

1/2 tsp salt

1 tsp coriander, ground

1/4 cup fresh cilantro, chopped

Instructions

1. Heat up oven to 400°F.

2. Add every ingredient into a big bowl and toss until chickpeas and cauliflower are completely coated.

3. Prepare an aluminum foil lined baking sheet.

4. Spread chickpea mixture on the prepared baking sheet.

5. Place baking sheet into the preheated oven and roast until softened, for about 25 minutes.

6. Serve and enjoy.

Roasted Beet Hummus

Preparation Time: 10 minutes

Cook Time: 0 minutes

Serves: 10 servings

Ingredients

8 oz. (roughly chopped and pat dried) roasted beets

1 (15 oz.) can (rinsed) chickpeas, no-salt-added

¼ cup olive oil

¼ cup tahini

1 garlic clove

¼ cup lime juice

½ tsp salt

1 tsp cumin, ground

Instructions

1. Add salt, cumin, garlic, lime juice, oil, tahini, beets and chickpea into a food processor and combine.

2. Puree mixture for about 2-3 minutes until a finely smooth consistency is reached.

3. Serve hummus with desired pita or vegetable chips.

Snacks and Nibbles

No-Dairy Turmeric Falafel

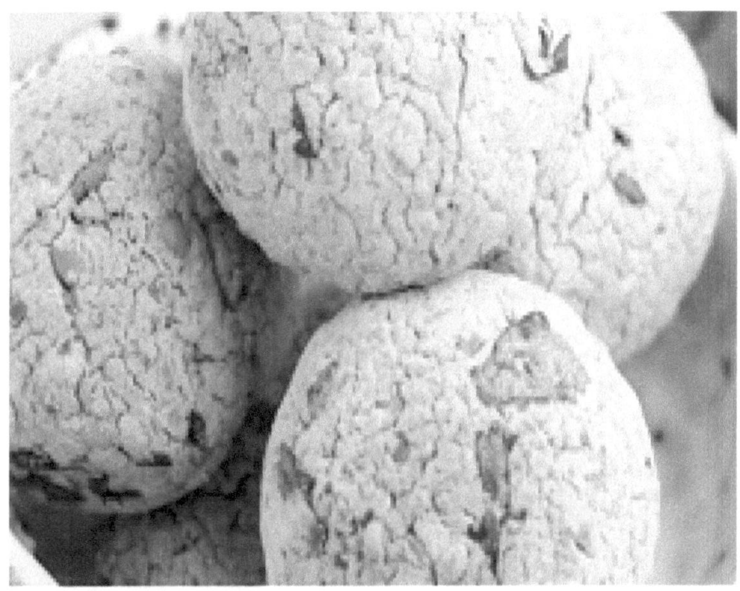

Preparation Time: 10 minutes

Cook Time: 20 minutes

Serves: 2 servings

Ingredients

2 tbsps aquafaba (chickpea liquid from the chickpea can)

1 (14 oz.) can chickpeas

1 garlic clove

1 handful fresh cilantro

1 tsp olive oil

1 tsp turmeric

Salt and pepper, as needed

Instructions

1. Heat up oven to 390°F.

2. Add every ingredient into a food processor or a high speed electric blender.

3. Process until a smooth consistency is reached.

4. Make blended batter into balls using clean hands.

5. Bake balls in the preheated oven for 20 minutes.

6. Serve and enjoy.

Walnut Almond Truffles

Preparation Time: 10 minutes

Cook Time: 0 minutes

Serves: 12 servings

Ingredients

1 cup almond flour

1 cup (soaked for 2-3 hours in water and drained) walnuts

1/4 cup cocoa powder

3/4 cup (soaked for 1-2 hours in water and drained) organic raisins

1 teaspoon lime zest

3 tablespoon maple syrup

Instructions

1. Add drained walnuts into a food processor and process until finely grated.

2. Add almond flour into the processor and process until evenly distributed, for 1 minute.

3. Pour flour mixture into a bowl.

4. Add raisins into the empty food processor and process until finely chopped.

5. Add maple syrup and cocoa powder into the food processor while it runs and keep blending until a very smooth consistency is reached.

6. Add the flour mixture into the food processor and process until incorporated.

7. Pour mixture into a bowl and form into 3/4" balls.

8. Place bowl into a refrigerator.

9. Serve and enjoy.

Curry Lemon Nuts (No-Sugar)

Preparation Time: 5 minutes

Cook Time: 20 minutes

Serves: 2 cups

Ingredients

1 1/2 tbsps coconut oil

2 cups (walnuts, pecans and cashews) or preferred mixed nuts

1 tbsp curry powder

3 tbsps fresh lemon juice

Salt, as needed

1 tsp turmeric powder

Instructions

1. Heat up oven to 350°F.

2. Add turmeric powder, curry, lemon juice and coconut oil into a big bowl and combine.

3. Add nuts into the bowl, toss and stir until well combined.

4. Season nut mixture with salt.

5. Prepare a parchment paper lined baking sheet and add the seasoned nut mixture.

6. Place baking sheet inside the preheated oven and bake for 10 minutes.

7. Stir nut mixture and bake until nuts are toasted, for 5-10 more minutes.

8. Let sit until cooled, serve and enjoy.

Almond Cherry Chocolate Clusters

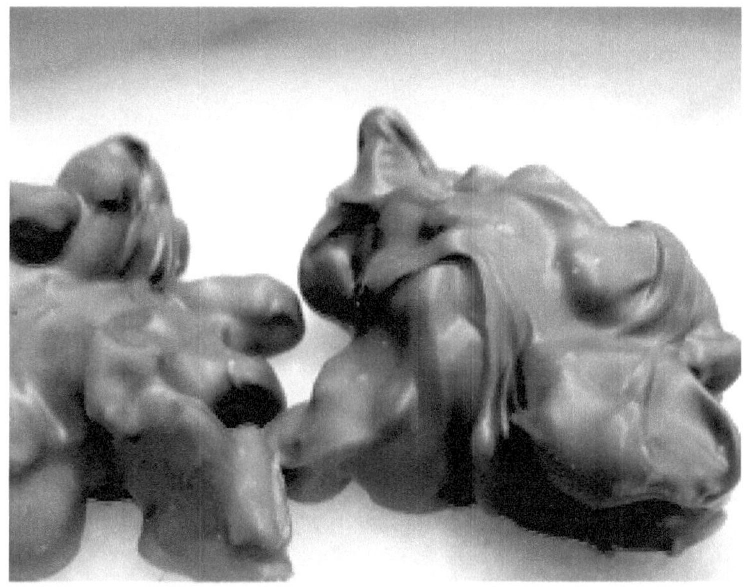

Preparation Time: 10 minutes

Cook Time: 5 minutes

Serves: 12 chocolate clusters

Ingredients

1/2 cup (roughly chopped) dried cherries

1 cup (roughly chopped) almonds, toasted

6 oz. finely chopped dark chocolate

Instructions

1. Add cherries and almonds into a fairly big bowl and toss until combined.

2. Prepare a wax paper lined baking sheet.

3. Add half of the chocolate into a double boiler top over the lowest heat and just simmering water.

4. Stir chocolate often and ensure that the water does not touch the pan at the top.

5. Take out chocolate with top pan from the double boiler and add the remaining chocolate half.

6. Stir chocolate mixture until combined and let sit until cooled.

7. Get rid of the simmering water in the underside of the double boiler and replace it with fresh tap water that is warm.

8. Put the melted chocolate pan over the one with warm tap water.

9. Add the nut mixture into the chocolate and stir until incorporated.

10. Scoop out a generous tablespoon of the chocolate mixture onto the prepared baking and leave room of about 1" between each cluster.

11. Transfer baking sheet into a refrigerator for 15 minutes until set.

12. Serve at room temperature.

Crunchy Almond Cranberry Granola Bars

Preparation Time: 20 minutes

Cook Time: 35 minutes

Serves: 1 serving

Ingredients

1 cup crispy brown rice cereal

3 cups rolled oats, old-fashioned

½ cup (toasted & chopped) almonds

1 cup cranberries, dried

¼ tsp salt

½ cup (toasted & chopped) pecans

½ cup smooth almond butter

1/3 cup brown rice syrup

1 tsp vanilla extract

Instructions

1. Heat up oven to 325°F.

2. Prepare a 9x13" parchment paper lined baking pan and coat lightly with cooking spray.

NOTE: Use surplus parchment paper, so that it hangs over 2 sides of the pan.

3. Add salt, pecans, almonds, cranberries, rice cereal and oats into a big bowl and combine.

4. Add vanilla, almond butter and rice syrup into a saucepan over med-heat.

5. Stir to combine and heat for 1 minute.

6. Add rice syrup mixture into oats mixture and stir until well distributed and combined.

7. Pour oat mixture into the prepared baking pan and press well with the back end of a spatula.

8. Place baking pan into the preheated oven and bake for 30-35 minutes until firm in the center and the edges are golden brown.

9. Let sit for 10 minutes until cooled before lifting out of the baking pan.

10. Place on a cutting board and cut into twenty-four bars.

11. Let sit until wholly cool for about 30 minutes, before separating into bars.

12. Serve and enjoy.

Walnuts and Apricots

Preparation Time: 3 minutes

Cook Time: 0 minutes

Serves: 1 serving

Ingredients

7 walnut halves

5 apricots, dried

Instructions

1. Add walnuts and apricot into a bowl.

2. Toss until combined and pour into a resealable snack container.

3. Enjoy.

Scrumptious Dark Chocolate Trail Mix

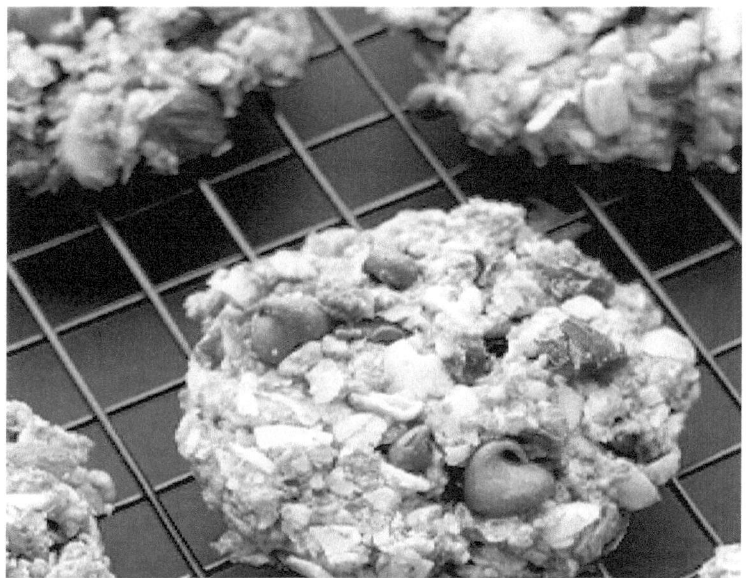

Preparation Time: 5 minutes

Cook Time: 0 minutes

Serves: 1 serving

Ingredients

4 apricots, dried

2 tbsps whole almonds

2 tsps dark chocolate chips

Instructions

1. Add chocolate chips, apricot and almonds into a bowl.

2. Mix until well combined.

3. Serve and enjoy.

Soup

Lentil Lime Soup

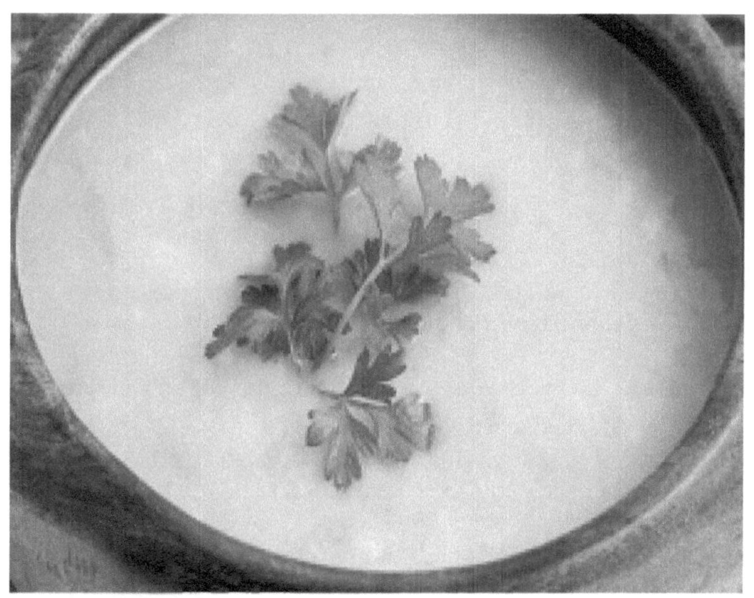

Preparation Time: 5 minutes

Cook Time: 1 hour 30 minutes

Serves: 8 servings

Ingredients

1 diced yellow onion

1 tbsp olive oil

1 1/2 cups celery, diced

1 1/2 cups carrots, sliced and diced

3 minced garlic cloves

1 tsp salt

2 1/2 (32 ounces) boxes vegetable broth

4 tsps ginger, fresh grated

2 cups (rinse & get rid of stones by picking) green lentils

2 tsps turmeric, dried

3 small limes, juiced

1/2 lime, zested

Instructions

1. Add oil into a big stock pot over med-heat.

2. Add salt, celery, carrots and onion into the hot oil and saute for about 5 minutes until tenderized.

3. Add ginger and garlic into the pot and saute for 1 more minute.

4. Add lentils, turmeric and broth into the pot and adjust heat to low-heat.

5. Simmer lentil mixture for 45 minutes, covering partially.

6. Add lime juice and zest into the soup and stir until incorporated.

7. Cook for 30 more minutes.

TIP: Pour in additional broth, if necessary.

8. Serve soup and enjoy.

Veggie Lentil Soup

Preparation Time: 20 minutes

Cook Time: 1 hour 30 minutes

Serves: 8-10 servings

Ingredients

4 cups yellow onions, chopped

1 lb. dry French green lentils

3 minced garlic cloves

4 cups leeks, white part only (chopped)

1 tbsp kosher salt

1/4 cup extra-virgin olive oil

1 tbsp fresh thyme leaves, minced

1-½ tsps black pepper, freshly ground

3 cups celery, diced

1 tsp cumin, ground

3 qts. chicken stock

3 cups carrots, diced

2 tbsps red wine vinegar

1/4 cup tomato paste

Parmesan cheese, freshly grated

Instructions

1. Add just enough boiling water to cover and the lentils into a bowl and soak for 15 minutes.

2. Drain off water.

3. Add cumin, thyme, pepper, salt, olive oil, garlic, leeks and onions into a big stockpot over med-heat.

4. Saute until veggies are softened and translucent, for 20 minutes.

5. Add carrots and celery into the pot and saute for 10 more minutes.

6. Add lentils, tomato paste and chicken stock into the pot and place lid over pot.

7. Bring mixture to boiling.

8. Adjust heat and simmer soup until lentils are well cooked, for 60 minutes without covering.

9. Check for seasoning, adjust as necessary and pour in the red wine.

10. Sprinkle soup with freshly grated parmesan and drizzle with olive oil.

11. Serve and enjoy.

Sweet Potato and Roasted Red Pepper Soup

Preparation Time: 25 minutes

Cook Time: 30 minutes

Serves: 6 servings

Ingredients

2 chopped medium onions

2 tbsps extra-virgin olive oil

1 can (4 ounces) diced green chiles

1 jar (chopped, with the liquid reserved) roasted red peppers

1 tsp salt

2 tsps ground cumin

3-4 cups sweet potatoes, peeled & cubed

1 tsp ground coriander

2 tbsps fresh cilantro, minced

4 cups vegetable broth

4 ounces (cubed) cream cheese

1 tbsp lime juice

Instructions

1. Add olive oil into a big soup pot over med-high heat.

2. Add onion into the hot oil and cook until tenderized.

3. Add coriander, salt, cumin, green chiles and red pepper into the onion mixture and cook for 1-2 minutes.

4. Add the vegetable broth, sweet potatoes and the reserved roasted pepper juice into the pot.

5. Bring mixture to boiling.

6. Adjust heat to med-low and place lid over pot.

7. Cook for 10-15 minutes until the potatoes are softened.

8. Add the lime juice and cilantro into the pot and stir until combined.

9. Let soup sit until slightly cooled.

10. Puree soup until desired consistency is reached, using an immersion blender.

11. Cook soup until warmed through.

12. Season with salt and serve.

Potato Curry Soup with Roasted Cauliflower

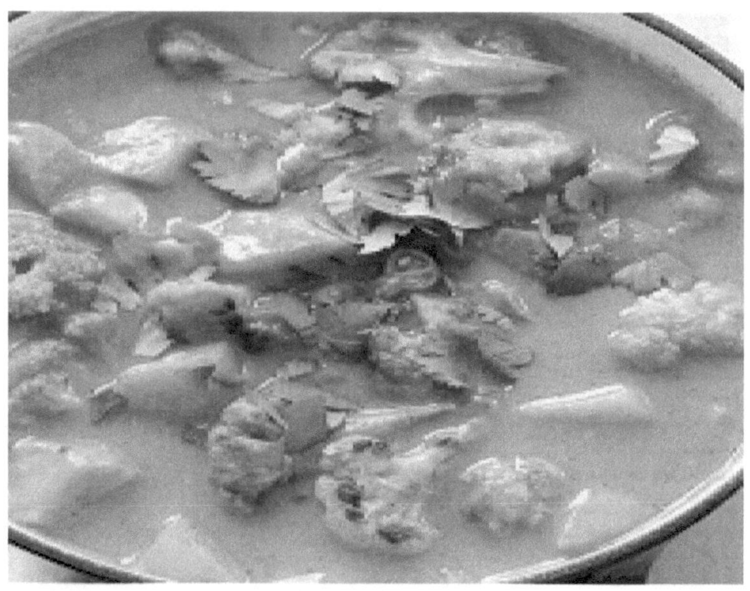

Preparation Time: 50 minutes

Cook Time: 1 hour

Serves: 8 servings

Ingredients

2 tsps cumin, ground

2 tsps coriander, ground

1½ tsps turmeric, ground

1½ tsps cinnamon, ground

¾ tsp pepper, ground

1¼ tsps salt

1 (cut into small florets) small head cauliflower

1/3 tsp cayenne pepper

1 chopped large onion

2 tbsps (divided) olive oil

1 cup carrot, diced

White Onions

1½ tsps fresh ginger, grated

3 minced large garlic cloves

1 (14 oz.) can tomato sauce, no salt added

1 fresh (minced) red chile pepper + more for garnish

3 cups russet potatoes (peeled & cut to 1" dices)

4 cups vegetable broth, low-sodium

1 (14 oz.) can coconut milk

3 cups sweet potatoes (peeled & cut to 1/2" dices)

2 tbsps lemon juice

2 tsps lemon zest

Instructions

1. Heat up oven to 450°F.

2. Add cayenne, pepper, salt, turmeric, cinnamon, cumin and coriander into a small bowl and mix.

3. Add cauli-florets into a big bowl, drizzle with 1 tbsp oil and toss until covered.

4. Sprinkle 1 tbsp cayenne mixture over cauli-florets and toss until covered.

5. Transfer the coated cauli-florets onto a rimmed baking sheet in one layer.

6. Place baking sheet into the preheated oven and roast for 15-20 minutes until cauliflower edges are browned.

7. Remove cauliflower from the oven and let sit until needed.

8. In the meantime, add the remaining 1 tbsp olive oil into a big pot over med-high heat.

9. Add carrot and onion into the hot oil and stir cook for 3-4 minutes until beginning to brown.

10. Adjust heat to med-heat and keep cooking for 3-4 minutes until the onion is tender, while stirring continuously.

11. Add the remaining cayenne mixture, chile, ginger and garlic into the big pot and stir cook for one additional minute.

12. Add tomato sauce into the pot and stir while simmering for a minute.

13. Add lemon juice and zest, sweet potatoes, russet potatoes and broth into the pot.

14. Place lid over pot, adjust heat to high and bring mixture to boiling.

15. Adjust heat to low, simmer mixture for 35-40 minutes, until veggies are softened, stirring mixture every now and then while pot is partially covered.

16. Add roasted cauliflower and coconut milk into the mixture and stir until evenly distributed.

17. Simmer mixture until heated through.

18. Serve soup garnished with chiles and cilantro.

19. Leftover can be placed in a refrigerator for up to 5 days.

Turmeric Ginger Carrot Medicinal Soup

Preparation Time: 5 minutes

Cook Time: 15 minutes

Serves: 2 servings

Ingredients

1 (peeled & chopped) parsnip

4 (peeled & chopped) carrots

4 (crushed) garlic cloves

1 (coarsely chopped) yellow onion

3 cups warm vegetable broth, low sodium

2 tsps coconut oil

1" (peeled & grated) ginger knob

1 tsp turmeric powder

Pinch cayenne pepper

1/2 of a lime, juiced

Serve with

Coconut flakes

Black sesame

Greek yogurt

Fresh parsley

Instructions

1. Heat up oven to 350°F.

2. Prepare a parchment paper lined baking sheet.

3. Add garlic, onion, parsnip and carrots into the prepared baking sheet and season with cayenne and turmeric.

4. Drizzle baking pan mixture with coconut oil and toss until wholly coated.

5. Place baking pan into the preheated oven and roast for 15 minutes.

6. Pour roasted mixture into a high speed electric blender.

7. Add ginger, lime juice and veggie broth into the blender and puree until a creamy and smooth consistency is reached.

8. Split soup into bowls, garnished with coconut flakes, sesame, fresh parsley and Greek yogurt.

9. Serve warm and enjoy.

Thai Pumpkin Soup

Preparation Time: 5 minutes

Cook Time: 7 minutes

Serves: 4 servings

Ingredients

4 cups veggie or chicken broth

2 tbsps red curry paste

1¾ cup coconut milk (reserve 1 tbsp coconut milk for garnish)

2 (15 oz.) cans pumpkin puree

1 (sliced) large red chili pepper

Garnish with

Cilantro, optionally

Instructions

1. Add curry paste into a big saucepan over med-heat and cook until the paste is aromatic, for about 1 minute.

2. Stir in the pumpkin and broth into the saucepan and cook until soup is bubbly, for about 3 minutes.

3. Add coconut milk into the soup and cook for about 3 minutes until hot.

4. Scoop soup into bowls, garnished with sliced red chilies, cilantro and the remaining coconut milk.

Spiced Lentil Soup

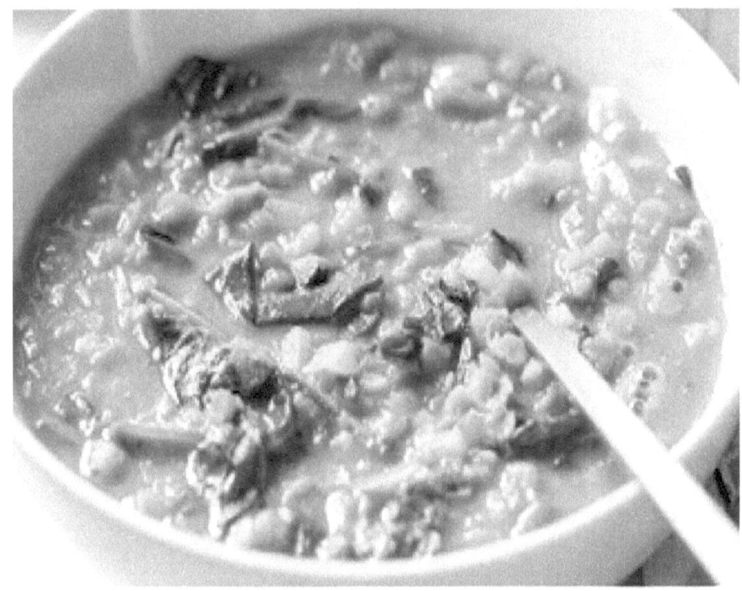

Preparation Time: 15 minutes

Cook Time: 20 minutes

Serves: 7 cups

Ingredients

2 cups onion, diced

1 1/2 tbsps olive oil

2 tsps turmeric, ground

2 large minced garlic cloves

1/2 tsp cinnamon

1 1/2 tsps cumin, ground

1 (15 oz.) can diced tomatoes, with juices

1/4 tsp cardamom, ground

3/4 cup (rinsed & drained) uncooked red lentils

1 (15 oz.) can coconut milk, full-fat

1/2 tsp fine sea salt

3 1/2 cups vegetable broth, low-sodium

Cayenne pepper, as needed

Freshly ground black pepper

2 tsps fresh lemon juice

1 (5 oz.) package baby spinach

Instructions

1. Add garlic, onion and oil into a big pot.

2. Add a pinch of salt into the garlic mixture and stir until incorporated.

3. Saute mixture until onions is tenderized, for 4-5 minutes over med-heat.

4. Add cardamom, cinnamon, cumin and turmeric into the pot and stir until combined.

5. Keep cooking until aromatic, for 1 more minute.

6. Add generous amount of pepper, salt, broth, red lentils, coconut milk and diced tomatoes with juices into the pot.

7. Add cayenne pepper into the pot and stir until combined.

8. Adjust temperature to high heat and bring mixture to a low boil.

9. Adjust heat to med-high once boiling, and simmer soup without covering until lentils are softened and fluffy, for 18-22 minutes.

10. Remove pot from heat, add spinach into the soup and let sit until wilted.

11. Add lemon juice into the soup and stir to combine.

12. Check for seasoning and adjust pepper and salt as necessary.

13. Scoop soup in serving bowls and serve with lemon wedges and toasted bread.

Turmeric Ginger Coconut Soup

Preparation Time: 5 minutes

Cook Time: 10 minutes

Serves: 4-6 servings

Ingredients

1¾ cups coconut milk, full-fat

1 qt. vegetable or chicken broth

½ tsp ground turmeric

A knob of (peeled & sliced very finely) fresh ginger

¼ tsp cayenne pepper

1 lime, juiced

2 tsps coconut oil

A handful of (coarsely chopped) cilantro

Sea salt and freshly ground black pepper, as needed

Instructions

1. Add every ingredient into a fairly big saucepan over med-heat, excluding the coconut oil and cilantro.

2. Bring mixture to a gentle simmer, and keep simmering for 5-10 minutes.

3. Take saucepan off heat and let sit for some minutes until cooled.

4. Generously sprinkle black pepper and sea salt over soup.

5. Add coconut oil and cilantro into the soup.

6. Check for flavors and add more lime juice if desired.

7. Serve soup and enjoy.

END

Thank you for reading my book.

Leslie Phillips

9 781719 345712